AGAINST ALL ODDS

AGAINST ALL ODDS
How to Move from Provider-Centered Care to
Patient-Centered Care
Copyright © 2014 by Ruth A. Tarantine, DNP, RN

Disclaimer: I have tried to re-create events, locales, and conversations from my memories of them. In order to maintain anonymity, I have changed the names of individuals and places; I may have changed some identifying characteristics and details, such as physical properties and places of residence. This book is not intended as a substitute for the medical advice of physicians. The reader should regularly consult a physician in matters relating to his or her health or the health of a loved one, particularly with respect to any symptoms that may require diagnosis or medical attention.

To contact the author, Ruth Tarantine, visit:

Book website.............. : www.HealthCareAgainstAllOdds.com

Book inquiries............. : Info@HealthCareAgainstAllOdds.com

Email .... : Ruth@HealthCareAgainstAllOdds.com

LinkedIn..................... : http://www.linkedin.com/in/ruthtarantine

Facebook .... : https://www.facebook.com/
HealthCareAgainstAllOdds

Eldercare
Navigators, LLC .... : www.ElderNavigators.com

Printed in the United States of America

To contact the publisher, inCredible Messages Press, visit
www.inCredibleMessages.com

ISBN 978-0-9889266-5-3 Paperback

ISBN 978-0-9889266-6-0 e-Book

Book coach.............. : Bonnie Budzowski, inCredible Messages, LP

Cover design............ : Bobbie Fox, Bobbie Fox, Inc.

Cover photograph.... : Dan Tarantine

Timeline illustration.. : Catie Tarantine

AGAINST ALL ODDS

HOW TO MOVE
FROM
PROVIDER-CENTERED CARE
TO
PATIENT-CENTERED CARE

Ruth A. Tarantine, DNP, RN

DEDICATION

This book is dedicated to my parents, who taught their children that *love* is a verb.

CONTENTS

PREFACE III

ACKNOWLEDGEMENTS VII

TIMELINE IX

FIND YOUR POWER IN A BROKEN SYSTEM 1

BE FULLY PRESENT AND FULLY INVOLVED AS A FAMILY 27

ADVOCATE FOR QUALITY OF LIFE— AS YOUR LOVED ONE DEFINES IT .. 43

INSIST ON PATIENT-CENTERED CARE 67

NAVIGATE A BROKEN HEALTH CARE SYSTEM 91

MOVE SUCCESSFULLY ACROSS THE CARE CONTINUUM 109

NAVIGATE INSURANCE, MEDICARE, MEDICAID, AND VA BENEFITS 137

DEAL PRODUCTIVELY WITH ANGER AND FRUSTRATION 165

SAY GOOD BYE AS YOUR LOVED ONE AND FAMILY CHOOSE 183

ONE YEAR LATER 199

APPENDIX A: THE PATIENT'S BILL OF RIGHTS 205

APPENDIX B: SERIOUS REPORTABLE EVENTS 209

REFERENCES AND KEY SOURCES 213

ABOUT THE AUTHOR 221

PREFACE

I WROTE THIS BOOK FOR SEVERAL REASONS. As a nurse of twenty-five years, I thought I knew what patient-centered care was. I believed I delivered patient-centered care to my patients. I followed the rules in the hospitals where I worked and, again, I believed those rules were based on having the patient at the center of care. I had worked at numerous facilities across the United States, and care delivery was, and is, largely the same.

It wasn't until my family embarked on a serious health journey with my mother that I realized that the U.S. health care system was designed to deliver care with the provider at the center. Little did I know that the journey with my mother would serve to challenge my beliefs and provide me with more education in 2½ years than in all my years at any institution of higher education combined. Although there is an anomaly here and there, I learned through experience and research that provider-centered care is the norm throughout the United States.

If you are a patient or a family member of a patient, I wrote this book, for you first. My goal is to make your journey throughout this nation's health care system easier. Further, I want to help you ensure that you or your loved one receives the quality of care that allows the highest possible quality of life—according to the patient's own definition. It's the patient's and family's definition of *quality of life* that matters, not the provider's, insurance company's, or even mine. I became a nurse to help others and, if this book helps one patient or family, I have done my job.

In addition to sharing my family's journey with Mom's health care, this book presents the results of the extensive research I conducted on topics relevant to patients and families. I've developed practical tools and compiled resources in each area. Although my family was determined to care for my mom at home when at all possible, I realize that at-home care isn't realistic or desirable for all families. I've tried to provide information that allows you to chart your own path. You'll find tools ranging from documents to guide your family in difficult conversations about end-of-life wishes to checklists to help you choose the best long-term care facility.

In addition, I wrote this book because many doctors and nurses asked me to. One nurse told me she witnessed a new type of patient-centered care with our family. Ironically, we never thought about our approach because our mother and her wishes were always at the center of our decisions. We assumed all families had the same expectations.

Many doctors commented on our ability to push the boundaries of Medicare to approve customized care for Mom. The doctors couldn't believe that, given her complex medical challenges, my mom was surviving *against all odds*. Again, we didn't think twice about asking for care modifications; Mom deserved the modifications, and we knew they saved the health insurance company, Medicare, and Medicaid money. Obviously, they realized it, too.

In sharing this story, I hope to increase awareness and start conversations with direct patient-care providers.

Every individual who makes an effort toward patient-centered care makes the world a better place for all of us.

Finally, I wrote this book to honor my mom, Ruth E. Tarantine. Mom was heartsick when she witnessed families suffering over their frustration in navigating the health care system on behalf of their loved ones. Mom insisted that I share with others what I learned from my family's experience. At first, I did this in hospital waiting rooms. Then my brother Rick and I founded our company, Eldercare Navigators, LLC. Before her death, Mom helped design the logo, which is a compass.

This book is a tribute to my mother's strength, perseverance, and compassion. It is a way in which she is still reaching out to help others—to help you. Nothing would make her happier.

Welcome to the Tarantine family journey. More important, welcome to the lessons and resources compiled from our journey to make yours easier.

Acknowledgements

To those doctors and nurses who encouraged me, thank you. To the small team of physicians who collaborated with us until the end to provide my mom the quality of life she desired, I am grateful.

Mom's PCP, Dr. Farrell, and his partner, Dr. Barrett, deliver patient-centered care every day. So do specialists Dr. Santini, Dr. Belista, and Mary, RN. I hope you and your loved ones are lucky enough to have providers like them in your final days.

I thank Bonnie Budzowski of inCredible Messages. Bonnie coached me through the book-writing process from start to finish. She tirelessly edited the manuscript, and I am convinced she is the only person outside my family who knows my Mom's journey as well as we do. She was always sensitive to the loss I suffered, and I will be forever grateful.

I acknowledge Julianna Onofer, who reviewed the book for the readability of content. Sometimes a third-party edit helps you explain the content better.

Pieces of the book came together because of others. The timeline of my mother's illness was made possible by Catie Tarantine. She was called to rescue me when my version of the timeline became *frozen in time*. Of course, Catie completed it in one evening.

I also want to thank Rick Tarantine, Esq., who performed a legal review of my book. All names and places were changed to promote anonymity and to reinforce that this story can take place at any hospital in any town, in any state. The U.S. health care system and its deficiencies have no boundaries—status or wealth can't protect you from it.

Dan Tarantine took the cover photograph. This picture of my Mom, in Dan's Corvette, is timeless. It has proved repeatedly that one picture can have a huge impact on another's perception. This picture gave Mom's life meaning to providers while in the hospital, and it continues to give her life meaning in death.

Last, and certainly not least, I want to acknowledge my siblings: John and his wife, Elaine; Kathy; Dan; Rick and his wife, Debbie; and Bob and his wife, Pam. Despite the miles between many of us and the length of time between visits or conversations, we know we can count on one another in times of need. They say it takes a village. I'm not so sure about that. All you need is a few committed individuals who were taught that *love* is a verb.

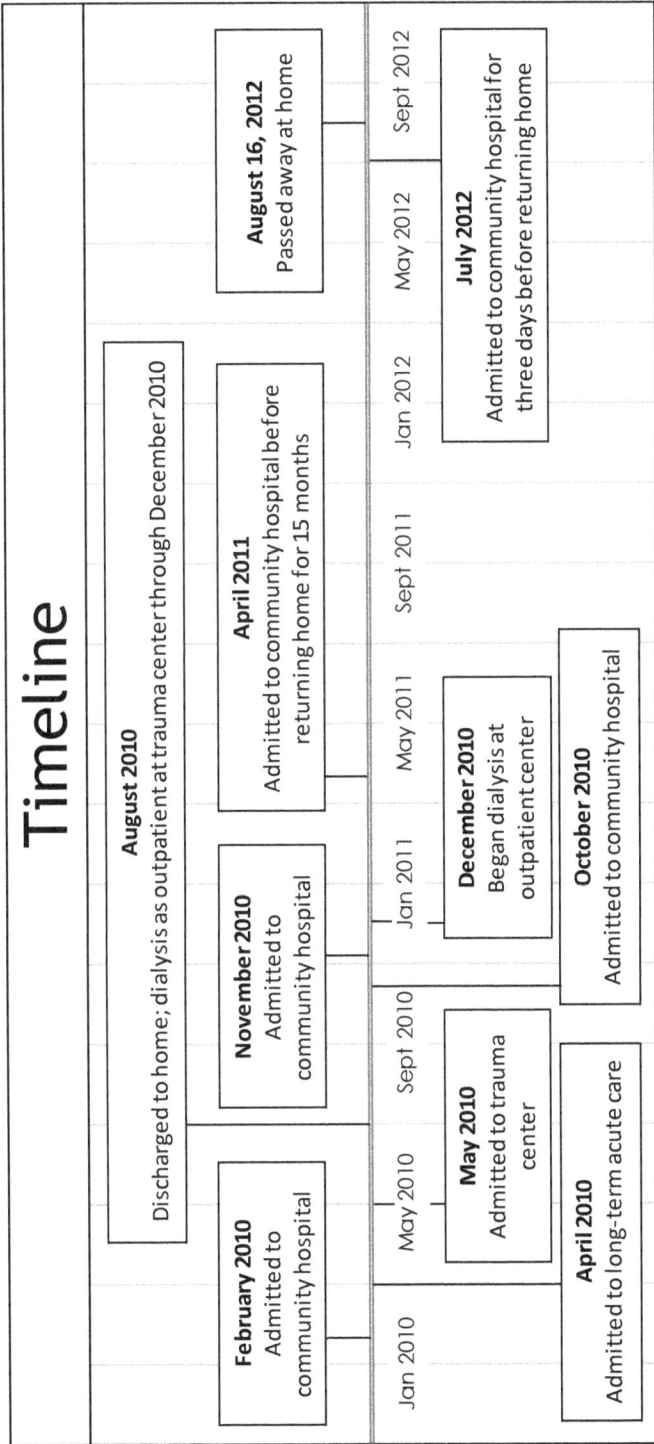

Timeline

February 2010
Admitted to community hospital

May 2010
Admitted to trauma center

April 2010
Admitted to long-term acute care

August 2010
Discharged to home; dialysis as outpatient at trauma center through December 2010

November 2010
Admitted to community hospital

December 2010
Began dialysis at outpatient center

October 2010
Admitted to community hospital

April 2011
Admitted to community hospital before returning home for 15 months

July 2012
Admitted to community hospital for three days before returning home

August 16, 2012
Passed away at home

Jan 2010 May 2010 Sept 2010 Jan 2011 May 2011 Sept 2011 Jan 2012 May 2012 Sept 2012

CHAPTER 1

FIND YOUR POWER IN A BROKEN SYSTEM

> *Family means no one gets left behind or forgotten.*
>
> ~ David Ogden Stiers

"ARE YOU READY TO SIGN THE CONSENT FORM for your mother's operation?" asked Dr. Johns, the fourth-year surgical resident. Barely 30 years old, he glanced up from his clipboard.

"I am," I uttered as I reread the surgical consent form for the tenth time.

"I know you're aware that your mother is very sick. We don't know what we'll find once we open her up, but at her age she is at very high risk for many complications, including death," Dr. Johns droned as if reciting a script committed to memory.

"I am aware of that, Doctor, and although my mother is 81 years old, she has a terrific quality of life. She still drives, shops, goes to church, and makes huge Sunday dinners for the family. In fact, we just got back from a cruise to the Bahamas a few weeks ago."

"Well, we have to talk about your mom's code status in case something happens," Dr. Johns stuttered nervously. "We have to talk about whether or not to revive your mom if something goes wrong."

Without hesitation, I answered, "Mom is full code. She and I have talked about this, and she wants everything done to save her life."

"I understand what you are saying," responded the doctor, "but your mother is 81 years old and very sick. Even though she was independent before she got sick, she is 81. Do you think she would want to be kept alive by artificial means if something happened?"

Mom's choice to be full code meant that, if something should happen in the operating room or afterward, the doctors would be obligated to try everything possible to save her life. The doctor was implying that, because of Mom's frailty and age, the chosen plan of action was inappropriate. He was suggesting that under the circumstances Mom might prefer a no-code, or do-not-resuscitate (DNR), status.

"I know my mother's wishes," I responded. "We talked about it, and full code is her wish. Despite her age, she has a great quality of life. Just look at her Facebook site."

The look on the doctor's face changed. "Her Facebook site? Really? Are you kidding? Your mother has a Facebook site? I don't even have a Facebook site," he said, surprised.

"Mom has a Facebook site. In her profile picture, Mom is behind the wheel of a Corvette."

"Wow, she must be a really active 81-year-old if she has a Facebook site. I can understand why you want everything done. Okay, I just marked in her chart that your mother is a full code," Dr. Johns proudly stated.

I stood briefly paralyzed, unable to hide my disbelief while trying to comprehend this conversation with the doctor who held my mother's fate in his hands. He was the surgical team's designee, the person charged with interpreting the wishes of the family and patient. Here was a young, 30-something resident determining that my mother's life now had value because she had a Facebook account.

I remember thinking, "Is he serious? Surely he can't think that Facebook equates with high quality of life?" Apparently, Dr. Johns did think this, as evidenced by the quick conveyance to his peers the information that my mother had a Facebook account. All of a sudden, my 81-year-old mother became *cool* and talk of her Facebook account became normal conversation at bedside rounds every morning.

At this point, I realized I had entered what I now consider the parallel universe of health care. This universe is clearly broken and, on behalf of my mother, my entire family needed to become actively involved in it. Her very life depended on it.

EVERY FAMILY HAS POWER

The encounter with Dr. Johns is just one of many bizarre encounters experienced during my family's 2½-year journey with my mother through the health care system. Along the way, we won a number of skirmishes to ensure Mom got the care she deserved, the highest quality of life possible under the circumstances, and the services and financial support to which she was entitled. We honored my mother's life and end-of-life wishes, even in the face of recurring problems and persistent opposition. My mother's case was a first in a number of contexts. For example, she was the first patient with a tracheostomy in the state of Pennsylvania to receive hemodialysis at home. I'll explain the meaning of these terms as our story unfolds.

After spending numerous hours in various family waiting rooms in a variety of hospitals and encountering countless roadblocks, my family members realized our experiences were not atypical. In fact, the frustration, confusion, and fear we experienced were themes common to all families. We saw those feelings in people's faces and overheard those feelings in their conversations. We tried our best to help. Now that Mom is gone, I have a message and strategies to share with families who are currently in waiting rooms and in the throes of an acute or long-term illness of a family member.

All families have power in health care and, with some guidance, you too can take charge of your family member's care. Although it may seem daunting, as though you are in a parallel universe in which you don't speak the language, you can win battles on behalf of your parent, life partner, child, or other loved one. You can turn love into action that gets the results your loved one needs. Even if your loved one passes away, you rest assured, knowing that you did everything possible to surround your loved one with love, dignity, and comfort in his or her final days.

Because I am a nurse and my brother is an attorney, it may seem as though our family had unique advantages in our situation. My brother and I, however, know it wasn't our professional expertise that helped our family—because the health care system itself is broken. Things in health care don't necessarily proceed in a linear or logical fashion. Our family experienced as many moments of heartbreak, frustration, and confusion as any other family. The ingredients that led to success are ones every family has: presence and persistence.

I recall lying on a cot next to my mother's bed during week 2 of her hospital stay. It was about 2 a.m., Mom was getting sicker, and the doctors didn't know why. I was talking on the telephone to my brother Dan, who lives in Phoenix. Dan could sense my despair and fear through my tears. He ended the conversation with words I will never forget, "Don't worry, Little Sister; the cavalry is on its way." Although I already had the support of two brothers, Rick and Bob, who lived in Pittsburgh, the three of us were exhausted between working and hospital visits. Within seventy-two hours, Dan was in Pittsburgh, along with my sister, Kathy, from Seattle, and my brother, John, from Atlanta. We all came together to formulate and implement TARP: the Tarantine Assistance Recovery Plan.

LIKE EVERY STORY, MOM'S WAS COMPLICATED

My mother suffered, late in life, from adult-onset asthma of unknown cause. There were times when she was admitted to the hospital to receive steroids and antibiotics. She was also a tightly controlled diabetic who followed doctor's orders and was actively involved in managing her health. Mom had decreased kidney function due to diabetes, but her condition was stable. Her kidneys were able to meet the needs of her body.

On a New Year's cruise to the Bahamas in 2009, I noticed Mom was showing the beginning signs of breathing problems. I began to pay attention, thinking it might

soon be time for another hospital visit. These periodic
visits had become normal for Mom; it seemed she required an annual tune-up.

Things unraveled unexpectedly on February 9, 2010,
and I called the ambulance during a record-breaking
snowstorm. Mom was rushed to the community hospital
where I happened to work at the time. Mom was in severe respiratory distress.

The journey that began that night would eventually
involve a series of surgeries, medical errors, and complications that took place in a number of different hospitals
and facilities. Although my mother's initial reason for
hospitalization was asthma, she soon developed a gastrointestinal problem and needed exploratory surgery. The
surgery was complicated, and Mom was sent to the
Intensive Care Unit (ICU). She was on a ventilator—that
is, a machine that forced air into her lungs by means of a
tube down her throat.

Because of the asthma, weaning Mom off the ventilator was difficult. After a number of days, doctors performed a tracheostomy—they made a small hole in
Mom's windpipe and inserted a tube into her neck so she
could breathe. The goal of the tracheostomy was to help
wean Mom off the ventilator. In Mom's case, the trach
became semi-permanent. Mom then needed frequent
suctioning through her tracheostomy to remove mucus
from her lungs, to help her breathe. This became a com-
plicating factor in her health care.

In March of 2011, roughly one year after Mom's
original hospital admission, one physician labeled my
mother as one big *iatrogenic cascade*. An iatrogenic
cascade is a series of adverse events caused by medical
personnel or procedures or that develops through expo-

sure to the environment of a health care facility. Many of
the things that happened to my mother are what the
National Quality Forum, a nonprofit health care standards organization, calls never events. A *never event* is an
inexcusable serious mistake that should never occur in a
health care setting.

During the 2½-year journey, my mother suffered a
number of adverse medical events. In an *adverse medical event,* a patient is injured as the result of a medical
intervention, not as the result of an underlying medical
condition. An adverse medical event is any aspect of
health care management that causes unintentional harm
to a patient. It is fair to say that all never events are adverse events, but all adverse events are not necessarily
never events. The worst of Mom's never events was a
stage IV bedsore (pressure ulcer).

A bedsore occurs when an area of skin breaks down
because something keeps rubbing or pressing against it.
Since a bedsore is preventable with proper patient moni-
toring, a bedsore is considered a never event. A stage IV
bedsore is one that has become so deep that there is
damage to muscle and bone. Mom developed a stage II
bedsore during her first week in the ICU. Because the
bedsore wasn't properly treated, it progressed to stage IV.
A stage IV bedsore is a painful, chronic wound that cannot be healed, only managed. Mom's bedsore was a
source of severe pain and discomfort until the day she
died.

Mom also suffered from multiple hospital-acquired
infections (HAIs). The infections included hospital-
acquired pneumonia that she never got rid of, in spite of
recurring treatment over a two-year period. The antibiotics used to treat this pneumonia killed Mom's remaining

kidney function, requiring her to be on hemodialysis for the rest of her life. Although Mom had suffered renal insufficiency from her diabetes, she didn't progress to renal failure and require dialysis until she acquired an infection at the community hospital. From then on, Mom needed hemodialysis three times a week. Hemodialysis is a type of dialysis in which the circulating blood is filtered through a machine with an artificial kidney. Bodily waste products that are normally excreted through the urine are removed in the process.

Soon after Mom's initial hospital admission, as specialist after specialist was added to her case, communication between providers and family became increasingly difficult. It didn't take long before our family realized that someone had to be with Mom at all times. Although my mother knew her medications and disease processes and asked many questions, she was too sick to keep track of everything that was happening. I could tell she was becoming scared.

As a nurse, I wanted to be able to reassure her. I wanted to believe that the health care system worked and would deliver quality care to my mother. I wanted to trust my peers and the organization I knew so well. I knew that the nurses and doctors caring for Mom were competent and skilled. I knew they wanted to provide the best care possible, but that wasn't enough.

I also knew that medical errors happen to patients at every hospital, in every city, despite the best efforts of health care providers. Doctors and nurses provide care in a maze of broken processes. As a daughter, I began to watch my mother fall victim to the broken health care system that reports more than 98,000 deaths per year due to medical errors (Committee on Quality of Health Care in America [CQHCA], 1999). My mother was rapidly becoming a statistic, and my family had to intervene.

Nothing along this journey was easy. Our journey began with continuously defending my mother's wishes to remain a full code. Then she received the tracheostomy and was on a ventilator. After two months in the community hospital, Mom was transferred to a long-term acute care (LTAC) facility that specialized in weaning patients from ventilators. Although Mom made progress weaning from the ventilator during the month she was in LTAC, her progress was interrupted.

Mom lost consciousness one day when staff members were moving her from a chair back to bed. Because of this, Mom needed to be transferred back to a hospital that provided acute care. Our city's trauma center was the closest hospital, so we had her taken there.

After one month in the trauma center, we tried to get Mom transferred back to the LTAC facility that had been caring for her when she had lost consciousness during the move to bed. The insurance company denied the transfer back to LTAC because, before her hospitalization, Mom had failed to wean in the time allotted. Mom's physicians told us that research showed that an 81-year-old woman in my mother's condition would not come off the ventilator. Ironically, neither the physicians nor the insurance company was able to show us this research.

We were told that my mother would have to leave the hospital and go to a nursing home. There she would receive care but not rehabilitation. What the providers said didn't matter though, as my mother had already decided what she wanted, and our job was to advocate for her. Mom wanted to get better, or at least have a chance to get better. Our job was to ensure she got that chance.

Every week we had a family meeting at the hospital, with the doctor du jour, the nurse manager, case manager, and ancillary personnel (specialists in respiratory, physical, occupational, or speech therapy). In these meetings, we were repeatedly told that we had to make a decision about where to place Mom. Every week, my family had the same response. Mom was coming home—period. They all thought we were crazy. My past experience told me otherwise.

VIEWING ILLNESS FROM A DIFFERENT ANGLE

When I was a new nurse, I worked as a liver transplant nurse at the same trauma center that cared for my mom. Transplant nursing is unlike any other specialization. Nurses care for patients who are the sickest of the sick. They care for patients and families who realize that every moment is a blessing. Transplant families understand that life will never be perfect, so they take what they can get. If that means being discharged from the hospital to a hotel room (because you are from out of state) with a feeding tube, multiple drains, and an IV pump, you'll take it. For a transplant patient, quality of life is about seizing the window of opportunity when discharge is possible. That window is when you are infection-free and your immune system is strong enough to battle potential threats. Quality of life is about giving patients a glimmer of hope in the storm.

My mother was no different. She wanted a quality life, and we wanted that for her. We knew we had to seize that window of opportunity whenever it came. Our family believed Mom would be most comfortable and most likely to heal at home. Her children and extended family members were prepared to move mountains to make that happen. We would learn what we needed to learn and combine our energies and strengths to provide whatever Mom needed.

I knew we would encounter many obstacles in trying to get my mother home. I knew also that it would be possible if someone dared to challenge the way things had always been done. Eventually, we were told that taking my mother home with a tracheostomy would be the easy part. Dialysis would be our barrier. Due to outpatient dialysis center criteria, patients with a tracheostomy cannot be dialyzed at an outpatient center. This meant that Mom could only be dialyzed at a hospital or nursing home. We were told that we could not take her home.

We felt like we were fighting a losing battle. We had to find physicians and nurses who thought as we did. We had to find providers who were capable of thinking beyond *That's the way we've always done it.* We had to focus on what we could possibly change and ignore everything else. Taking my mom home was our primary objective, and all of our energy had to be spent on making sure this happened. The insurance company, a crucial player at this stage of the game, would remind us that we were pushing the envelope.

We constantly communicated with providers and the insurance company, to remind them of our goal as well as the fact that we weren't going away—we weren't going to give up. We didn't give up. We brought Mom home, complications and all. She lived every minute fully and died on her own terms.

Obviously, not every patient or family believes that caring for a loved one with a severe illness at home is ideal. You may think the choices we made were extreme. That's okay. The point is that your loved one and your family get to decide what *quality care* and *quality of life* mean to you. Know each other's wishes; know each other's strengths. Advocate for what you want and what you believe is best for your loved one and your family.

OUR SECRETS TO SUCCESS WILL WORK FOR YOU

After six months in health care facilities (two hospitals and one LTAC facility), Mom was discharged to go home with a ventilator and eventually became Pennsylvania's first person with a tracheostomy and ventilator to receive home hemodialysis. Although she had periodic hospital admissions after that, at one point in her 2½-year journey, she was home and out of the hospital for fifteen consecutive months. Every physician and nurse involved with her care for any length of time was amazed at Mom's resilience and spirit. Those physicians and nurses told me I had to write this book. Those providers said that, in my mother's case, they had witnessed a new type of patient-centered care.

Looking back, I attribute our family's success to relentlessly following specific guidelines:

1. Be present.
2. Know your loved one's wishes.
3. Expect the health care system to be broken.
4. Insist on communication.
5. Insist on patient-centered care.
6. Learn to speak in dollars and cents.
7. Take care of yourself.

These practices are powerful—and they are available to any family.

1. BE PRESENT

Each of our family members realized that being present at my mother's bedside was the single most important factor that could proactively drive her care. Ask any nurse or physician about family presence at the bedside. He or she will agree that it makes a difference.

Family members do not need to have medical or legal knowledge to advocate for their loved ones. They just need to be there. Families ask questions, press for answers, and want their loved ones to receive good care. They can be persistent. The bottom line is that patients with families at the bedside receive more attention from health care staff. Being present, both physically and mentally, on a journey through the health care system is something any family can do. The degree of family involvement will vary, depending on whether family members live near the patient or have other obligations, but one thing is certain: Their involvement will make a significant difference in the care their loved one receives.

When my mother was a patient on the medical surgical floor, my family was there twenty-four hours a day. We took shifts. I would arrive at 8 a.m. to hear rounds, and a sibling would relieve me in the afternoon. Another sibling would spend the night on a cot in my mother's room. When my mother was in the ICU at the trauma center, in her room we had a calendar with the names and shifts written so my mother knew who was coming every day.

Not every family can be present all the time, especially during daylight hours. These families can still make their presence known and be involved in their loved one's care. Technology can often offer out-of-town family members the ability to be present in the care of their loved one.

As a nurse, I have participated in health care provider–family meetings where the family was calling in via Skype. FaceTime (via Apple technology) is also a wonderful tool for out-of-town family members to communicate.

This book represents a toolbox of sorts that families can open at any time. You'll find a variety of tools to help your presence with your loved one be effective. Chapter 2 will describe our family's experience and provide practical suggestions that all families can follow. For example, I'll share the detailed template I used to create a binder that allowed me to organize Mom's medical information and keep track of discussions with doctors, commitments from staff, and test results. This binder was invaluable as we advocated for Mom.

2. KNOW YOUR LOVED ONE'S WISHES
    Long before my mother's illness, she discussed with the rest of the family her wishes regarding life and death. We knew how Mom defined *quality of life,* how she felt about being kept alive via artificial means, and how she felt about organ donation.

    Mom gave us the priceless gift of communicating her wishes. We were forced to make some extremely difficult decisions over our 2½-year journey, but making them was much easier because we knew we were honoring Mom's wishes. My mother made it clear that as long as she had her mind, as she put it, she wanted to live. She had her mind right up to the end; in fact, she didn't hesitate to share a piece of her mind with various doctors along the way.

In addition to family discussions, various tools are available to help you and your loved ones communicate regarding issues surrounding health care and the end of life. My mother designated me the durable power of attorney concerning health care. However, she also insisted that all of her children agree to any major health decision, so the burden wouldn't be solely upon me. Chapter 3 of this book, which is about quality of life, will discuss the issues and describe the tools available to you.

3. EXPECT THE HEALTH CARE SYSTEM TO BE BROKEN

As a medical professional, I know that health care workers are good people who try to deliver quality care. I know also that health care in the United States is far from perfect. In fact, in 2000, the World Health Organization ranked the United States 37th in health care quality (Murray & Frenk, 2010). For a variety of reasons, medical errors happen to patients at every hospital, in every city, no matter the education or concern of providers.

Official organizations have launched a number of initiatives for change, many of which are becoming increasingly tied to compensation for health care facilities. Change in entrenched systems, however, occurs slowly. Meanwhile, mistakes continue to threaten the safety of patients. My mother's stage IV bedsore was caused by a failure of communication in the electronic medical record as well as provider inattention to standard protocols. The hospital-acquired infections were caused by hygiene failures. Mom also suffered from ICU psychosis, which involves an altered mental status caused by the unnatural environment of an ICU. ICU psychosis is preventable. In my mother's case, ICU psychosis was exacerbated by missed medications.

In another mistake, a bone infection in my mother's bedsore wound was missed for months because no one bothered to read the full report of a scan. And one day I found Mom lying in a hospital bed with no identification band on her body. I recall thinking, "This is why people die in hospitals."

I learned to expect the health care system to be broken. I stopped being shocked by failures in systems and practices. I kept my binder with all Mom's information—including test results, consults, and plan of care—with me at all times. My family members and I asked more and more questions. When something didn't seem right, we pressed until we located the problem.

Chapters 3 and 4 outline national efforts to improve health care, including the drive toward patient-centered care and the safety goals of the Joint Commission, the organization that accredits more than 20,000 U.S. health care organizations.

4. INSIST ON COMMUNICATION

When a patient enters a hospital, doctors order consults from various specialists to assess and treat the patient effectively. Soon after Mom's initial admission, as specialist after specialist was added to her case, communication between providers and family became increasingly difficult. In fact, I began to worry that communication among doctors was becoming so difficult that no one was effectively managing Mom's care.

As a nurse, I knew that poor communication plays some part in most medical errors. I considered my mother fortunate that Dr. Farrell had been her primary care physician (PCP) for over twenty-five years. Dr. Farrell and his partners knew my mother and family well, and they were proactive in communicating the plan of care with my mother and the family.

One day, after I came to the staggering realization that 39 health care providers could potentially write orders concerning my mother in any given week, I decided to have a conversation with the PCP. One of Dr. Farrell's partners, Dr. Barrett, was rounding that day.

"Dr. Barrett, may I ask you a question?" I asked respectfully. I didn't want to offend the doctor. I had known him for a long time, and I knew he paid very close attention to his patients.

"Sure, Ruth, what is it?" he answered, turning to make eye contact.

"Who is coordinating my mother's care? I'm not sure who is driving the bus, so to speak," I said as I smiled.

"Well, that would be the primary care group. That would be Dr. Farrell and me," he said.

"Well, there seem to be some things falling through the cracks. Every time I ask one of the specialists a question, I get a different answer. Everyone is on a different page. Do you know how many doctors are seeing my mother?" I asked.

"A lot. I know we have many consults written. We're not quite sure what is going on with your mother yet, so there are a lot of doctors involved. Would it help if we called you in the morning and updated you? I will be seeing your mother for the next four mornings. I don't mind," said Dr. Barrett.

"Thank you. That would be great," I replied.

Dr. Barrett called me the next morning, and he called me every morning that he made rounds that included my mother. I would normally receive a call from either him or Dr. Farrell between 6 and 6:30 a.m. Next to my bed, I kept a tablet with my questions, and I used the tablet to make notes from our conversation, since I was often asleep when a doctor called.

Two weeks after asking Dr. Barrett about care coordination, I was in my mother's room when Dr. Barrett rounded. He told me that he had given our conversation a lot of thought and wanted to apologize. He said he realized that they weren't coordinating care as well as they should have been. If an attentive, proactive PCP has an initial lapse in care coordination, what is happening in cases with less than ideal PCPs?

Although good communication is essential at every step in health care, it is critical during times of change or transfer between facilities. For example, when a patient transfers to a long-term acute care (LTAC) or rehabilitation facility, that facility will get a summary of the hospital stay. The facility will rely on family members to communicate more fully. This seems crazy, especially in an era of electronic records, but it is true. I discuss our experiences with communication in detail throughout this book. The guidelines in Chapter 6, which cover movement along the care continuum, will be especially helpful to families.

5. INSIST ON PATIENT-CENTERED CARE

In the United States, according to long-standing practice, a patient entering a health care facility gives up control. Patients are relegated to the role of recipients rather than partners in healing practices. This practice hinders the healing process and creates emotional distress for the patient.

The basic definition of *patient-centered care* is this: Nothing about me without me. In other words, patient-centered care involves the patient in the planning and implementation of his or her care.

Many of the roadblocks our family encountered were based on the entrenched practices in provider-centered care. These practices included everything from inconvenient visiting hours to extra days in the hospital, based on inappropriate rules. Every time we came up against the phrase *That's the way it's done*, we knew we were butting up against provider-centered care.

Throughout this book, I describe our battles to receive patient-centered care. For example, I discuss how we pursued acupuncture treatment for Mom in the ICU, and how, when she finally received it, hospital staff crowded the door because the event was a first in the ICU.

In many cases, you won't get patient-centered care unless you pursue it relentlessly. With perseverance, however, you can get exceptions to hospital and insurance practices so you can customize your loved one's care and improve his or her quality of life. Be present. Ask questions. Speak up. Keep good records. Learn to think beyond *how it is always done*. Refuse to be intimidated. Most important, don't give up.

6. LEARN TO SPEAK IN DOLLARS AND CENTS

In the early weeks of July 2010, we were involved in a drawn-out battle with the Medical ICU in the trauma center. Each week, in the meeting our family had with health care providers, we reiterated that we would not place my mom in a nursing home. We were determined to take her home.

On this particular day, Dr. Daniels changed his typical answer. "You can take her home today if you want. I'll write the orders," he smiled. "She's only on the ventilator at night to rest. The problem isn't the vent, the problem is with dialysis," he stated.

The case manager, Missy, chimed in, "He's right. We'll never find a place to dialyze her as long as she has the tracheostomy. No outpatient center will take her. Outpatient centers can't dialyze trach patients. We've run across this before. That's why she has to go to a nursing home."

I responded, "She's not going to a nursing home. Dr. Daniels just said that she can go home with the vent. This health system owns several hospitals. Are you telling me that not one of them can dialyze her? I am sure you can make it work if you want to. We'll take her wherever we have to for dialysis."

"It's not that easy," Missy said, "A hospital has to have an outpatient dialysis license in order for your mother to be dialyzed there. The only hospital out of all of the hospitals in the health system that has an outpatient license is this hospital, and I don't know if the dialysis administrators would agree to do it. I doubt it."

"Why wouldn't they? Would they rather she stay in the ICU instead?" I questioned. "Because she isn't going to a nursing home."

"You're going to have to accept that your mom needs to go to a nursing home, Ruth. I'll ask the manager of the Dialysis Unit, but don't get your hopes up," Missy stated, obviously annoyed.

I left the meeting that day feeling optimistic. Although I didn't personally know the manager of the Dialysis Unit, I knew she had worked in the unit for over thirty years. I also knew that she had a long history of dealing with patients who were outliers. This hospital had an outpatient license because it dialyzed many of the international patients who came to our city for transplants. The hospital also dialyzed a handful of homeless patients whom other centers wouldn't accept. Would they agree to accept my mother?

The insurance company balked at our idea of taking Mom home until we emphasized what the discharge to home would mean to the company. My mother, who was costing the hospital and the insurance company money, would be discharged. The insurance company would have to pay for the medical equipment that she would need at home, but it owned the medical equipment company. The family would be providing the care at no cost. In our weekly hospital meetings and our conversations with the insurance company, we kept talking in dollars and cents. Finally, the idea clicked. Financially, taking Mom home would be a win for the insurance company.

I am not sure when all of the involved parties spoke to one another, but I do know that suddenly everyone was on board with the plan to allow my mom to go home. The logistics of dialysis fell into place. Mary, the manager of the Dialysis Unit, agreed to dialyze my mother as long as I signed a paper agreeing to be responsible for my mother while she was at dialysis. Mary wanted family with Mom and tending to certain needs, since Mom was more complicated than the typical outpatient.

Now hospital personnel had a financial stake in getting Mom out of the ICU. The research that reported that an 81-year-old patient could not be weaned from a ventilator went by the wayside, and they started aggressively weaning my mother. My mother left the trauma center on August 23, 2010, without requiring a ventilator. We had the ventilator at home in case my mom needed it, but she never needed it after her initial discharge.

We were able to take Mom home because of Mary, who was willing to provide patient-centered care in an unconventional manner and because we persisted in speaking in dollars and cents until the insurance company finally heard our argument in terms that mattered to the company. You, too, can learn to speak in dollars and cents as you advocate for your loved one.

7. TAKE CARE OF YOURSELF

When a loved one is ill, every member of the family feels the strain. In addition to the emotional concern, you suddenly have countless more tasks added to each day and week. Although you want to be present for your loved one, you still have to go to work, maintain your household, and care for children. Add the challenges of dealing with a broken health care system, and you have a recipe for distress and anger.

You can imagine how I felt when a physician at a pain center vowed that the iatrogenic cascade, the domino effect of medical errors that my mother was experiencing, would stop under that physician's care. The doctor made that statement right before overdosing my mother with Neurontin, a medication that she failed to adjust for Mom's renal failure.

Throughout Mom's journey, I learned I could only give my best to Mom when I was taking care of myself and accepting help from others. As a family, we learned that caregivers do not typically burn out from providing direct care but from the avalanche of mundane life tasks, like grocery shopping, cleaning, and ordering medical supplies. We learned to accept help in these areas.

I describe our efforts at self-care in detail throughout the book. Chapter 8 focuses specifically on managing anger and frustration. This chapter also describes proactive survivorship, a health-supporting practice that helps families who have experienced medical tragedies and tragedies of other kinds to channel energy productively and honor loved ones.

THIS BOOK IS FOR YOU

The decision to write this book stems from the desire to help others who are battling the health care system themselves or on behalf of a loved one. I decided to write this book because I realized that the success we experienced with my mother's journey was not directly related to medical knowledge. At times, it may sound like it, but I assure you it wasn't. Much of what I learned came from families of patients whom I had cared for in the past. The recipe for success is rooted in the fundamental characteristics that we all have as humans.

Success was the result of navigating complex systems in which the rules are outdated and screaming to be challenged, and in systems in which rules can change, depending on who you speak to.

This book is designed to assist patients and families in navigating the broken health care system. You, too, can do this. Regardless of what the result needs to be, you can drive the care for you or your loved one to achieve that result. Whether your goal is returning your loved one to home, an assisted-living facility, or nursing home, the strategy is the same. I have organized the chapters based on themes that you will find repeatedly in health care.

The focus of this book is not only about what my family learned on this journey, it is about what we can share to lighten the load on your journey. The basic traits of the health care system that make it an inherently failed system are poor communication, lack of care coordination and cooperation between providers and families, and lack of transparency. Families have the right to expect communication, coordination, cooperation, and transparency from all providers. You will find tools within this book that will help you communicate your needs, wishes, and expectations to providers so you can navigate the broken health care system successfully.

CHAPTER 2

BE FULLY PRESENT AND FULLY INVOLVED AS A FAMILY

> *Hope is like peace. It is not a gift from God. It is a gift only we can give one another.*
> ~ Elie Wiesel

EARLY IN MOM'S ICU STAY at the community hospital, I walked into her room and found her wrists tied to the bed. This sometimes happens in an ICU, to prevent the patient from pulling out an essential tube or IV. The nurse told me Mom had pulled the breathing tube out of her throat. The staff had had to reinsert it. I then made a specific request that Mom's hands not be tied. I told the nurse I wanted to be called if Mom needed to be restrained; I would come in and sit with her to ensure she didn't pull anything out.

"Really?" the nurse asked, sounding surprised and genuinely concerned. "I've never had a family make that request before. It might happen at 3 a.m., and I would hate to call and wake you up. You need your sleep, too."

"I don't care what time it is," I shot back. "I don't want my mother waking up with tied hands. If she were sedated enough that she didn't know, it would be different, but I know the doctor doesn't want to sedate her too much because he wants to take out the breathing tube for good. I just can't imagine Mom waking up restrained, and I believe it only adds to her agitation."

That evening, the resident increased Mom's sedation with a short-acting medication, and Mom appeared to be comfortable and in a deep sleep when I left at 10 p.m. The phone rang at 4:30 a.m., with the nurse saying, "I hate to call you, but your mother is awake and trying to pull out her tubes. Her chart says you want to be called before we restrain her."

"I'll be right in," I responded. "Can someone sit with her until I get there? I won't be longer than thirty minutes."

I arrived by 5:15 a.m., requesting to see the resident who was covering my mother that night. He reported that, although my mother was doing fairly well with her breathing, the team was not planning to remove the breathing tube that morning. I asked if he could increase the short-acting sedation a little more to keep Mom comfortable, if they had no plans of removing the tube for at least twenty-four hours. The resident increased the sedation without hesitation. My mother was back to sleep within five minutes, and I was home in my own bed by 6:30 a.m.

This situation and others like it worried me. While patient safety always comes first, it just makes sense to try alternative methods before restraining a patient. Officially, restraints are used as a last resort. But this wasn't how the ICU was handling my mother's situation.

My presence and my insistence on a different approach made a huge difference in my mother's comfort level while she had the breathing tube. Families that are present and speak up make all the difference. You don't have to be in health care to suggest that caregivers take a different approach. You just have to be a human being who can imagine what it would feel like to be that patient. That's all.

It is safe to say my family was an anomaly in the way we defined being present for Mom. In fact, Mom expected one of her family members to arrive by 10 a.m. at the latest. Heaven forbid if we were late getting to the hospital.

We had two, possibly three, shifts each day of visiting Mom in the ICU. Usually, my sister, Kathy, took the first shift during the week. My brother Bob and his wife, Pam, took both shifts on Saturday, since Bob was on the road driving a truck all week. My brother Rick and his wife, Debbie, and I alternated weeknights and Sundays. Rick and I also attended every family-staff meeting, on Tuesday afternoons. My other brothers, John and Dan, flew home from Atlanta or Phoenix, respectively, to help when their schedules permitted.

When Mom was in the ICU, we were required to leave the hospital shortly after 9 p.m. However, when Mom was on a regular floor in the hospital, family members were present twenty-four hours a day. Someone was always in the room with her, unless nursing staff kicked us out for shift report. They eventually gave up on this.

Mom asked us to bring her calendar from home and hang it from her IV pole so she could easily see it from her bed. We filled in the schedule on a weekly basis, so Mom knew when each of her kids, in-laws, or granddaughter would be there. This gave Mom a sense of control. This gave her hope. We, her loved ones, gave her hope.

When a patient is in the hospital for an extended period, it's easy to give up all hope of recovery. My mother's initial hospitalization was a stay of just over six
months (from February 9 until August 23, 2010). She
spent most of this time in the ICU. During this time, we
did everything we could to be Mom's biggest cheerlead-
ers; in fact, we went as far as to buy pom-poms to cheer
her on as she worked to wean from the ventilator. Since
this weaning appeared to be the most significant barrier
to leaving the ICU, we supported Mom's efforts with
hope; encouragement; and, most of all, humor. Once
Mom could stay off the ventilator for twenty-four hours
at one stretch, she could be transferred out of the ICU.

In addition to the pom-poms, we bought a balloon
for every hour my mother extended her time off the
vent. Kathy purchased a reusable decal from the dollar
store that read "NO FEAR–NO LIMITS." She bought
plastic hands that clapped and lit up when you shook
them. Mom laughed. Before long, she used the clapping
hands to get staff members' attention.

Mom had family pictures all over her room. She also
had her favorite CDs. You could often hear Barbra Strei-
sand, Frank Sinatra, or Tony Bennett bellowing from
behind her closed glass door. As Mom progressed with
time off the vent, the room filled with more and more
balloons. At one point, she had 23 balloons and all of us
were cheering her on to go for the 24th. All Mom had to
do was stay off the vent for one more hour to receive her
final balloon.

It wasn't unusual for a staff member to walk past the
room and see one of Mom's family members jumping up
and down yelling a cheer with the pom-poms, encourag-
ing and motivating Mom to stay off the ventilator long-

er. I'll never forget the day I walked into the ICU and witnessed Dr. Goodwin, the attending physician, waving the pom-poms and cheering for the progress Mom had made the day before.

We pushed the limits on *normal family behavior* in the ICU. We wanted Mom to have as much control as possible. Having family with her all of the time helped to promote this. We wanted her to feel motivated and hopeful, so we celebrated every accomplishment, regardless of how small. The many balloons, pom-poms, and family pictures encouraged Mom and ultimately helped to engage the staff with our family.

At one point, Lisa, a member of the ICU management team, said to me, "You know, Ruth, I have never witnessed a family like yours. It has been a long road for your mom and family. I can see that nobody is giving up. I'll admit that the nurses had a hard time caring for your mom at first, because your family was always here. Now we all see what a difference your family has made in your mom's recovery. This experience has taught us all a lot."

Being present and involved in your loved one's care is essential, especially when any type of change is made. For example, when Mom was being transferred to the LTAC facility, we were given a 10-page document listing all of the facility's physicians. From this list, we were to choose the doctor who would care for my mom during her stay.

After choosing a well-known pulmonologist, I asked Denise, the patient liaison, for a schedule of dates and times of the family-staff meetings, so we could be sure to attend. Denise told me the doctor I had chosen didn't believe in having formal meetings. The doctor was willing to answer questions from the family as they came up, but she didn't have the time to meet with families.

"Well," I responded, "you might as well rip up the paperwork you just filled out and give me the list again. I certainly don't want a doctor who doesn't value the family as an integral part of the care team. If the doctor doesn't have time for us, she won't have time for my mother."

YOUR FAMILY AND COORDINATION OF CARE

Theoretically, a patient's primary care physician, supported by specialists, is the centerpiece and coordinator of care. Unfortunately, the system doesn't always work. The American Medical Association and federal government acknowledge there are gaps from lack of coordinated care. Donald Berwick, MD, former administrator, Centers for Medicare & Medicaid Services, has long advocated patient-centered care and the coordination of services to provide better quality and avoid duplication and waste. He lists the lack of care coordination as one of the top reasons for health care waste in this country (Berwick, 2004).

Being present and attentive is the most significant thing you can do to drive the care of your loved one. Your presence sets the tone for the care relationship you will develop during your loved one's hospital stay.

You do not need medical knowledge to make a difference. Simply pay attention to the care your loved one receives. Become comfortable asking questions. For example, you may notice your loved one is scheduled for a CT scan today, the same scan she had yesterday. Don't assume this is because the scan is needed. Assume that no one knows about yesterday's scan. Repeat testing happens frequently in a hospital. When you are in doubt about anything, ask questions.

In any given week, numerous providers have the potential to write orders regarding a patient, depending on how many specialists are consulted. Add to that number new residents and fellows who start rotations every month or two. A patient may have a totally new group of residents and fellows start midway through one hospitalization.

At every juncture along the health care journey, providers must communicate the plan of care to one another. With the number of people involved, you can imagine the opportunity for errors. In fact, the Joint Commission (2008) reports that 70% of errors reported to the commission are the result of poor communication, and many errors go unreported.

In most cases, especially complicated hospital admissions, only one person knows the patient's whole story, and that person is usually a family member. The actual patient is compromised by illness and will miss or misunderstand information.

When a patient transfers between care facilities, a family member usually provides the patient's medical history to the new facility. Although a verbal report is typically shared between facilities, providers choose to share only certain highlights to make the report succinct.

For example, when my mother was transferred from the hospital to the LTAC facility, the hospital sent a two-page discharge summary and a few thousand pages of medical records. Do you really think anyone read the thousands of pages? And not even the best doctor can summarize a complicated two-month hospital stay involving fifteen specialties in two pages. That's where our family stepped in.

I kept a notebook next to my phone so I could write things down during Mom's hospitalization. Sometimes I was called at 6 a.m. to give consent for a procedure. I would write down the name of the procedure, the name and spelling of the doctor's name, and the reason for the procedure. I didn't take a chance on memory. In fact, I organized a binder to keep an accurate account of Mom's health care encounters.

I had learned this approach from transplant families, who live and breathe their loved one's medical history. They keep journals, logs, and charts with lab and test results.

I learned that no news is *not* necessarily good news! I learned to request a copy of results of every diagnostic test for my binder. I learned that, if I didn't keep track of Mom's information, no one else would. Guidelines to create your own binder are included later in this chapter.

Organizing Your Family to Support Your Loved One

Undoubtedly, your loved one will receive better care if someone is there to help coordinate the care. Of course, families are diverse, with each member having unique strengths as well as limitations. When a loved one is sick, capitalize on each person's strengths.

During my mother's initial hospitalization, Dan proposed that we enact TARP, the Tarantine Assistance Recovery Plan. The plan outlined the areas where help would be needed after Mom was discharged, as well as how we would accomplish the goals of the plan.

I later learned that we followed the typical pattern of caregiving for families in the United States. My sister and I acted as the primary caregivers. Brothers Rick and Bob cared for Mom on the weekends. Brothers John, Dan, and Rick supplied the financial resources to hire additional nursing help. My sister-in-law, Debbie, cooked a big Sunday dinner every week—a dinner that provided leftovers to last the week. My cousin, Elise, sent several homemade meals to my house every month. While on break from college, my 20-year-old niece, Catie, cared for my mom.

Everyone was involved in some way, whether through direct care, dealing with legal affairs, cooking, running errands, doing laundry, or providing financial assistance. It was all equally important. Every job was vital to the success of the plan. No job or contribution was too small or insignificant.

Not everybody in every family is suited or comfortable providing direct care. That's okay because direct care duties are not the ones that typically cause caregivers to burn out. The combination of other duties—such as food shopping, cooking, laundry, cleaning the house, and ordering supplies and medications—often causes the burnout. Each family member *can* contribute, depending on his or her strengths. With careful planning, most responsibilities can be shared. One person doesn't have to bear the whole burden (financial, professional, or personal).

A study by the MetLife Mature Market Institute
(2010)—devoted to research on aging, longevity, and the
mature market—revealed interesting findings:

- The percentage of adult children providing
  personal care and/or financial assistance to a
  parent has more than tripled over the past fifteen years. Currently, a quarter of adult children, mainly baby boomers, provide these types
  of care to a parent.

- For a woman over 50, the total of wages lost
  due to leaving the labor force early because of
  caregiving responsibilities equals $142,693. The
  estimated impact of caregiving on lost Social
  Security benefits is $131,351. A very conserva-
  tive estimate of impact on the woman's pension
  is $50,000. Thus, the total cost impact of care-
  giving, on a female adult child who provides
  care to a parent, in terms of lost wages and Social Security benefits, is $324,044.

- For a man over 50, the total of wages lost due
  to leaving the labor force early because of
  caregiving responsibilities is $89,107. The esti-
  mated impact of caregiving on lost Social Security benefits is $144,609. Adding $50,000, a conservative estimate of the impact on the man's
  pension, the total impact equals $283,716 for a
  man.

- On average, then, the total average cost to a
  male or female, age 50+, who cares for a parent
  is $303,880.

- Children provide financial assistance to their
  parents, regardless of the children's gender or
  work status or the gender of the parents. How-

ever, men are more likely to provide financial
assistance than basic care.

I was surprised by these results at first. Then I realized the results described our family's circumstances.
When someone is caring for a loved one, he or she
doesn't necessarily think about future lost Social Security
benefits or pension dollars. Unfortunately, this is the
reality many caregivers face, and it will only become
worse as baby boomers age and need care.

Fortunately, many states are beginning to pay family
members to provide care to elders. Eventually, this will
become the norm, as boomers will exceed the number of
available caregiving options. Families will become the
solution to the pending caregiving quandary when the
aging baby boomers hit this nation's health care system.
This pending impact is being called the *aging tsunami* or
silver tsunami.

The MetLife study reinforces the overall financial
toll that caregiving can take on individuals and families.

ACTION STEPS FOR YOUR FAMILY

1. ### BE PROACTIVE: FORMULATE A PLAN
    Regardless of who is in the hospital, reach out to ex-
    tended family and friends for help. This is no time to
    be shy. Contrary to what you might think, family
    members and friends are usually eager to help and
    often just need clear direction. Be as clear as possible
    about what you need. Do you need someone to gro-
    cery shop? Take out your garbage? Pick up medica-
    tion or supplies? Babysit? Sit with a family member

when everyone else is at work? Let people know exactly what you need.

2. CREATE A SCHEDULE FOR HOSPITAL VISITS

Make it your goal to have someone present with your loved one for as many hours as possible. Since the goal is for your loved one to recover, he or she doesn't have to engage in conversation with every visitor. Just by being there, a visitor can reduce anxiety and promote rest for the patient.

For an extended stay, give your loved one a pocket calendar that shows the days and times visitors are scheduled. Provide telephone numbers in case the patient wants to ask someone to bring something. This may seem like overkill for the average hospital admission, but you never know when the average hospital admission will become, because of unanticipated complications, the nightmare hospital admission. Being prepared for the worst can often be the key to having a good outcome.

3. CARE FOR YOURSELF

If you happen to be the one visiting on many or most days, prepare for the long stay. Bring fresh clothes and hygiene products with you. Always have enough of your own medications. If, however, you are caught off guard and find yourself in another city or state without your medications, talk to your loved one's nurse about having a doctor write a prescription for you. Doctors are typically prepared to write prescriptions in these situations.

Make the effort to eat well, exercise, and take time for yourself. Locate the chapel or meditation room in the hospital. Use it to find quiet time to be alone with your thoughts. You will find the time alone, spent in prayer or meditation, to be crucial in maintaining your emotional and physical health. If you become sick, you won't be able to help your loved one.

4. BE DILIGENT ABOUT KEEPING GOOD RECORDS
    Health care is a maze, a world with its own set of rules and vocabulary. It is unrealistic to think you can navigate the maze without a map of where you have been and where you are going.

    Do not rely on your memory. When you keep good records, you'll have the information you need at your fingertips; you won't have to rely on hospital systems. You'll be prepared to fill in gaps in communication and coordination of care for your loved one. In addition, the health care providers will notice that you are writing everything down, from the procedure being ordered to the doctor who is ordering it.

    Follow the tips below to organize a binder to keep a record of your health care. Keep your binder with you at all times. You will see multiple specialists and receive results along the way. Keep these documents with you and refer to them when needed. You will be surprised and appalled at how many times you are the only one with the correct information.

    Most physicians, especially ones trying to manage the care between multiple providers, will embrace your binder. It will ultimately become a resource to make their job just a little bit easier.

5. ORGANIZE YOUR HEALTH CARE BINDER

A. Choose a heavy 1½ inch, three-ring binder.

B. Insert colored tab dividers (at least fifteen) and label them to make a section for information about:

- Each specialist
- Lab results
- Procedure and scan results
- Medications, herbal supplements, past medications, and doses
- Insurance and contact information
- Medical history
- Any research you have done
- Blank loose-leaf paper for jotting notes and answers to your questions

C. Use business-card pages and plastic sleeves to keep a record of the following:

- Every doctor you visit or consult
- Every lab or radiology department where testing is done
- Appointment-reminder cards
- Prescriptions and orders for future testing
- Any communication from a physician

D. Use CD holders to keep a copy of MRI or CT results. *Never give up your only copy of any test results.* If someone requests the results, ask the person to make a copy—staff members always can.

E. Include a calendar.
   - Choose or create a three-hole calendar.
   - Document the date of all tests on the calendar, so you can locate the date when needed.
   - Document dates on which you will need to call for appointments with physicians who will not let you schedule more than six months ahead.
   - Jot down comments on the sticky notes and use the notes to access key pages during appointments.

CHAPTER 3

ADVOCATE FOR QUALITY OF LIFE—
AS YOUR LOVED ONE DEFINES IT

> *Your perception is what determines your quality of life.*
>
> ~ Unknown

FROM NOVEMBER 2011, I HAVE a beautiful photo of my mother in my sunroom. The photo portrays a woman sitting contentedly in her wheelchair at a glass dining table. Mom is wearing a fluorescent yellow ball cap to block the rising sun as she reads her morning paper and drinks coffee. In the backyard is a deer feeder filled with 250 pounds of corn as well as a bird feeder full of exotic seeds. Mom made sure the animals were fed daily. She received great joy from watching herds of deer feed on the corn throughout the day. She could identify each of the brightly colored birds.

On the table in front of Mom sits a blooming Christmas cactus; a bud vase with a red rose; and a purple petunia, left over from summer, that refused to die. Also on the table is a bag valve mask (BVM) with an in-line suction catheter attached. This device provided manual ventilation via Mom's tracheostomy while Mom's lungs were suctioned. Beside the BVM is a nebulizer machine with aerosol medication attached. In the middle of all of this chaos is a fall centerpiece with the statement "Give Thanks." This was my mother's life.

Twenty months earlier, on March 24, 2010, soon after Mom was first admitted to the community hospital, a doctor wrote a note in my mother's medical record:

> Patient has a very poor prognosis for any meaningful recovery, in my opinion, given her continued MSOF [multisystem organ failure]—kidney/lungs/brain/heart.

Yet here Mom was in November 2011, sitting in my sunroom. Despite the doctors having told us there was no hope for recovery, Mom was enjoying life. What's more, she was at home rather than in a nursing facility. Many times during the previous twenty months, nursing home care was the best outcome doctors dared hope for.

We all have different definitions of *meaningful recovery*. We have different definitions of *quality of life*. My definition of *quality of life* has changed over the years. My mother's definition changed as well.

Every intern, resident, fellow, and all but one attending physician—Dr. Farrell, Mom's PCP—asked her the same question at various junctures, "If your heart were to stop, would you want everything done?"

My mother chose to be full code from the time she entered the hospital, meaning that whatever happened, she wanted every intervention to save her life. My mother replied the same way each time. She would look at me, roll her eyes, raise both hands in disgust, look back at the questioner, and answer, "Yes, why do you all keeping asking me this? I want everything done. Just because I'm 81 doesn't mean I don't want to be 82!"

The need to justify Mom's code status began on the first day and continued until she left the hospital for the final time. Once word spread of her Facebook account, however, the physicians backed off slightly.

In fairness to all doctors involved, they are required to ask patients about their code status. In asking the question, they are merely doing their jobs. However, asking a patient once should suffice. My mother often said, "If I were 40, they wouldn't be asking me this question 10 times." And she was right.

My mother was hospitalized initially for asthma. However, in roughly two weeks, she developed a gastrointestinal problem and needed exploratory surgery. The surgery was complex, and her recovery was complicated by multiple iatrogenic events, some that were never events. These events included the bedsore that developed during her first week in ICU and the hospital-acquired pneumonia in the second week.

Upon her admission to the hospital in 2010, my mother was a diabetic on insulin but not dialysis. Although she had some renal insufficiency from diabetes, her kidneys still functioned well enough to clear toxins from her blood. Hospital-acquired pneumonia, coupled with the antibiotics given to treat it, killed any remaining kidney function, causing renal failure. From that point on, Mom required hemodialysis. During most of her long illness, Mom needed a tracheostomy to breathe. Sometimes she needed the help of a ventilator also. The combination of tracheostomy and renal failure created all sorts of complications and challenges. Throughout it all, our family fought for Mom's right to have the least intrusive care and the highest quality of life possible.

What Is Code Status?

Code status is the term used by hospital staff to describe the procedures that can or will be performed on a patient if that patient's heart stops or lungs fail. When patients come into the hospital, they are automatically considered *full code* (all extraordinary medical interventions will be provided in the event of an medical emergency) unless patients provide instructions (oral or written) to stop these interventions from being performed on them.

Hospital personnel are required by law to ask all patients their preference about their code status on admission to the hospital. Two common code statuses are do not resuscitate (DNR) and do not intubate (DNI). Doctors may ask the following questions:

- If your heart stops, do you want us to use cardiopulmonary resuscitation (CPR) to try to bring back a normal heartbeat?

- If your lungs fail, which of the following options do you want?

   Option 1: To be connected to a breathing machine (requiring a breathing tube to be inserted into the throat, known as intubation) and have your underlying disease treated until you improve and can be disconnected from the machine to breathe on your own. If it becomes clear, after an extended period, that you are not likely to improve, the breathing machine would then be taken away and you would be allowed to die comfortably.

   Option 2: Not to be connected to a breathing machine under any circumstances, even if the doctors think they can treat your underlying condition. In this case, the hospital staff will make you comfortable and let you die without breathlessness or suffering.

Many hospitals also give patients a choice about whether to receive other treatments, such as feedings, fluids, antibiotics, electrical shock to the chest in case the heart beats too fast, ICU care, a pace-maker, and invasive procedures. These treatments can be discussed when you consider whether to have CPR, or they can be discussed and withdrawn, one at a time, if they are not working well.

Keep in mind that every hospital has its own guide-lines regarding code status levels.

For more information, see American Thoracic Socie-ty (2013).

A UNIQUE PERSPECTIVE ON QUALITY OF LIFE

As I mentioned in Chapter 1, I learned a lot from my experience working with transplant patients and their families. These families had no medical experience, but they were armed with the desire to give their loved ones some sense of normalcy and a better quality of life than a hospital can afford. I was involved with teaching spouses, parents, and friends of these patients how to empty drains, give medications, and deliver other nursing care that many believe can come with formal education only. Most of the family members were successful in caring for their loved ones.

These family members were present, both physically and emotionally, for their loved ones and were persistent in communicating their expectations. They kept a log of lab values, daily communications with providers, test results, and medication lists.

Transplant patients and their families taught me that anything is possible. They taught me that a health care provider's definition of *quality of life* doesn't matter. The only thing that matters is the patient and his or her wishes. Health care providers have the job of facilitating the patient's wishes.

I brought my perspective as a transplant nurse to my mother's situation. I never realized how much I had learned from those transplant families until my family was also involved in a long-term hospitalization of a loved one. The idea of seizing all the life you can grab meshed with Mom's desires. My siblings and I were willing to do whatever it took to take Mom home, even if her life would be far from perfect.

My siblings and I had to perform all the tasks cited on a long checklist before we were deemed competent to care for Mom at home. My family learned how to suction my mother through her tracheostomy, give meds through a feeding tube, change her bedsore dressing, and apply an ostomy bag. My sister, Kathy, and I each had to spend a night in the ICU, caring for Mom, to prove we could do all the typical ICU tasks. Kathy had worked in a lab; she had never provided direct care, but she learned how. My brother Bob, who came on Saturdays after driving a truck all week, had to demonstrate that he could care for Mom as well. The same held true for Rick, who came on Sundays. Even my 20-year-old niece, Catie, learned how to run the ventilator, suction my mother, give her feedings and meds via the feeding tube, and change her dressing.

All this competency testing took place in the weeks prior to us taking my mom home. In the process, Mom often joked that she might survive the hospital stay only to have one of her children kill her while trying to care for her. We did a lot of laughing while we were learning.

As evidenced by the photo of Mom enjoying her life in my sunroom, we did take Mom home. Home care

nurses and respiratory, physical, and occupational therapists visited the home frequently to ensure we were all
doing okay, but family members provided the most care.
For my siblings and me, some of the most precious and
memorable moments of our relationship with our mother occurred during the time we cared for her at home. I
still have spots of tube feeding on the ceiling in my
mother's bedroom. I'm not sure how it got there. Although my mother knew, she would never tattle on the
one who put it there.

Quality-of-Life Skirmishes

Although we cared for Mom at home, there were times
that she needed services in a health care setting. At one
point, while at the LTAC facility, Mom suffered an acute
hearing loss. She could hear on Wednesday but not
Thursday. When I walked into her room on Thursday
morning, Mom was petrified to the point of tears. Despite
using hearing aids in both ears, she couldn't hear me or
anyone else. "Ruthi," she mouthed (unable to speak because of the tracheostomy), "I can live with a lot of these
changes to my life, but I don't think I can live if I can't
hear. That's too much for anyone to bear. I have a trach,
a feeding tube, and dialysis. Now I'm deaf?"

My heart broke. I immediately asked Mom's nurse if
she knew about my mother's hearing loss. She told me
that she did and that she thought hearing loss was normal for Mom's age. I was upset. I said, "Normal hearing
loss occurs over a period of time. I know that some medications can cause hearing loss, but unless Mom received
medications I don't know about, medications can't be the

cause. Could you please call her doctor and ask for an ear, nose, and throat consult?"

The nurse was obviously irritated. She didn't see Mom's hearing loss as a priority. I saw it as the number one priority. My mother was scared. How was she supposed to participate in any form of rehab if she couldn't hear the directions? How was she going to work with respiratory therapy to come off the ventilator if she couldn't hear the directions? My mother was now isolated in a silent world. She already couldn't talk because of the tracheostomy, and now she couldn't hear either.

When the ear, nose, and throat (ENT) doctor came to assess my mother the next day, he couldn't find anything wrong and concluded the problem was just *old age*. I didn't agree with him. I asked for an audiology consult.

It was now Mother's Day weekend. John and his wife, Elaine, and Dan flew to Pittsburgh, and my mother spent the day with her six children, in-laws, and granddaughters. She was overjoyed. Despite her hearing loss and many other medical issues, she said it was the best Mother's Day she'd ever had.

The next day, however, my mother passed out when staff members were putting her back to bed after she had been sitting up in a chair for a few hours. Doctors weren't sure what caused the blackout. One doctor speculated that Mom might have had an irregular heartbeat.

My sister and I were with Mom that day. We knew that, in addition to having her deafness investigated, my mother needed a procedure performed on her bedsore and her dialysis catheter changed. We viewed these needs as an opportunity for her to go back to the closest hospital, a trauma center, to have everything done at once.

That afternoon my mother was transferred to the nearby trauma center and admitted to the Medical ICU. The ICU resident, Dr. Donlissen, prioritized her problems based on the traditional Airway-Breathing-Circulation (ABC) Model. This model reminds a practitioner of the priorities for assessment and treatment of patients in acute medical and trauma situations. Obviously, airway, breathing, and circulation are vital for life, in that specific order. Although I agreed with Dr. Donlissen's assessment, I let him know I was also concerned with Mom's acute hearing loss.

Dr. Donlissen informed me that hearing loss wasn't a priority. Hearing loss was outside the ABC Model, the model used for assessing patients. Despite my mother's fear and the impact hearing loss could have on her life, Dr. Donlissen dismissed the concern. I persisted and reminded him that it would be difficult for Mom to participate in her care if she couldn't hear and that hearing loss was a quality-of-life issue. He shook his head and said he would pass my concern on.

A few days later, another attending physician saw my mother and said that old age was the cause of Mom's hearing problem but that the physician would have an audiologist see her anyway. Fortunately, the trauma center was affiliated with an eye and ear institute. When the audiology intern, Dave, came to see my mother, he brought every tool imaginable. He eagerly performed a comprehensive assessment.

Despite two attending ENT physicians concurring that my mother's hearing loss was the result of old age, Dave's diagnosis was different. He found fluid behind both eardrums. Within fifteen minutes, the humbled attending ENT physician asked me for consent to perform a procedure to drain the fluid. The doctor made small slits in the eardrum, and the fluid drained out. My mother could hear immediately. So much for old age. I was happy; at the same time, I was saddened. How many other patients was this happening to? How many people must a family member ask before something is done? Hearing loss severely affected Mom's quality of life, but it wasn't a priority to anyone except her and her family.

At another point, my mother had been home for a few months and the tracheostomy had been recently removed. With the removal of her tracheostomy, Mom was able to transition to an outpatient dialysis center. During her first outpatient dialysis treatment, the technicians removed 1 liter of fluid. I knew my mother typically had 2 liters removed. I informed Bobbie, the nurse, of my mom's normal weight and that practitioners normally removed 2 liters of fluid during each treatment.

Bobbie, who didn't know my mother, said that she was going to err on the side of caution and limit the removal to 1 liter. Although I understood this rationale, I had been with my mother on this journey for almost eleven months. I knew how Mom responded to treatment and knew that 1 liter would not be enough. Mom reiterated to Bobbie that 1 liter would not be enough. The nephrologist, Dr. Michael, also knew this, but Bobbie refused to call Dr. Michael to verify. Instead, she made the decision to remove only 1 liter.

The following day, I found myself calling an ambulance at 6 a.m. My mother needed emergency dialysis. She couldn't breathe because of excess fluid in her lungs. When Mom arrived at the same community hospital where she was originally treated, Dr. Michael ordered a dialysis treatment. Unfortunately, since that hospital doesn't have a license to perform outpatient dialysis, they had to admit Mom. It was the day before her 82nd birthday.

Mom hadn't needed to be admitted for any medical reason; she had to be admitted because of a rule. Dr. Michael's hands were tied. The hospital had a license for inpatient dialysis only, so my mother had to be an inpatient. I was informed that her insurance company would not pay unless Mom was admitted.

My mother, who by this time had battled numerous hospital-acquired infections as well as other iatrogenic events, was being told that she would have to be admitted to the hospital because of a rule, not because she was sick. Common sense and cost were to be disregarded and the rule obeyed. I understood and appreciated the need for rules but couldn't rationalize this at all. My mother wanted to go home. She had spent enough time in the hospital that year and certainly didn't want to spend her birthday there as well.

After dialysis, Gerri, Mom's nurse, was admitting my mother to her room. I asked Gerri to call Dr. Farrell, Mom's PCP, to tell him we were leaving. Dr. Farrell was a longtime advocate of keeping geriatric patients out of the hospital. He would often tell my mother that the hospital was the most dangerous place for an elderly person. He would do everything possible to try to manage her asthma at home and only admit her if she didn't respond to treatment. Surely he would understand.

Dr. Farrell did understand, but the rules were the rules. He told Gerri to tell me that, if my mother left against medical advice (AMA), Mom would probably receive a bill for the dialysis. Even though there wasn't any medical reason for Mom to stay and no medical treatment would be administered after her dialysis session, the term *against medical advice* reinforced the rule that required her to stay.

I asked Gerri to get my mother the AMA form to sign and to notify Dr. Farrell that we would take our chances with billing. After all, the hospital system owned the insurance company. I knew the rules were the rules but, if Mom left the hospital, the hospital system and the insurance company would be saving money, right? Surely, someone could do the math.

We left the hospital. As I hoisted my mother's 5-foot–tall frame into my SUV, a huge smile flashed across her face. "The heck with them," she said. "I've spent enough time there. Are they crazy to think I would stay there when I am not sick?" We drove off as it started to snow.

My mother changed that night. She became empowered. She realized that she had control over her life again. And she never forgot her own power until the day she died. We never did get a bill for that emergency dialysis treatment at the hospital.

* * * * * * *

In April of 2011, long after the initial discharge and long after my mother's tracheostomy had been removed, she developed a dialysis-catheter infection and had to be hospitalized. During this hospitalization, Mom needed a simple procedure that was typically done on an outpatient basis. I was the only family member at the hospital when her vascular surgeon, Dr. Hada, called me on my cell phone. I remember picking up the phone and thinking how nice he was to keep me informed promptly.

Little did I know that my mother had just stopped breathing. Mom had experienced respiratory arrest when they tried to sedate her. The nurse anesthetist and anesthesiologist, both familiar with my mother and me, resuscitated her and had to place a tube down her throat and connect her to the ventilator so she could breathe.

Dr. Hada met me in the waiting room to update me on Mom's condition. He was visibly upset. He needed to know what I wanted done. I was alone at the hospital and couldn't make any decision like this by myself. I knew what Mom wanted. I also knew the severity of what had just happened.

In addition to being clear on her code status, my mother was also clear on something else. Any medical decisions that had to be made on her behalf had to be unanimous, with all six of her children agreeing. Although I was appointed the durable power of attorney and was the one Mom had designated to make medical decisions, she didn't want that burden to be on one person. My siblings in Pittsburgh quickly arrived at the hospital, and I phoned John, in Atlanta, and Dan, in Phoenix. We decided to continue to advocate for Mom's wishes, and she remained a full code. This happened on a Friday afternoon.

On Saturday morning, Mom was fully awake, alert, and asking for coffee and doughnuts. Dr. Santini, the pulmonologist, spoke to her and me at great length about having another tracheostomy inserted on Monday. He explained that this tracheostomy would allow us to take Mom home and suction her if need be. It would also allow her to use the ventilator at night, to rest. He advised us that this would be temporary and give her a chance to build up her strength.

When Mom agreed to have the tracheostomy, we had no idea she would receive great benefit and relief from this procedure, nor did we know she would have that trach for the rest of her life.

At this point, Mom moved in with me. She chose pink as the paint color for her new bedroom and a hydrangea border for the walls. She was happy to be alive.

REDEFINING *QUALITY OF LIFE*

I remember caring for Penny, a 40-year-old woman with no arms or legs, when I was in nursing school. Penny had developed a clotting disorder from an infection and had had to have her limbs amputated. I recall asking my nursing instructor, Mrs. Barnes, why anyone would want to live in that condition. Mrs. Barnes explained to me that people don't always get a choice. She said that Penny had adjusted to her new life and was happy she was alive. It took me years to understand what Mrs. Barnes told me that day. Often as a nurse, I watched patients and families adjust to a new normal, thankful for life.

Now my mother and family adjusted to a new normal. Mom and I developed rituals, such as the one we used when we had to make the hour-long drive to see Dr. Blackwell, the doctor who managed Mom's bedsore. I would pack a *go bag* full of medicine and medical equipment for the trip. Mom would look forward to a ride through the city, with a stop at the fast-food drive-through of her choice and a visit to my father's grave.

One day, on our way to see Dr. Blackwell, I stopped at a gas station to fill up. Opposite my SUV was a car with an elderly man pumping gas while his wife sat inside the car. Mom indicated that she needed to be suctioned. I grabbed the go bag and turned on the portable suction. I used the bag valve mask to give my mother some breaths mechanically and proceeded to insert the long catheter into her neck. The couple stared with eyes wide open. My mother and I started laughing uncontrollably. My mother, unable to talk because of the tracheostomy, mouthed the words, "I bet they don't see *that* every day!" She then pointed to a Kentucky Fried Chicken restaurant and mouthed, "Pull in. I want some popcorn chicken."

Eating—that was something directly related to quality of life that no one thought Mom could do while she had the tracheostomy. Initially, when discharged from the hospital in August 2010, Mom was sent home; care was to be provided by the hospital-owned home care agency. The agency sent a nurse and speech, physical, and occupational therapists to see my mother.

Mom so badly wanted to eat normally, but the speech pathologist was cautious. The therapist insisted that Mom eat a special diet, to avoid any potential of choking. Safety, rather than Mom's enjoyment of food, was the therapist's sole concern. Mom drank coffee thickened with baby cereal. Mom was not at all happy with the restrictions.

My family had grown up with my mom cooking big Sunday dinners. Now my sister-in-law, Debbie, had started cooking the Sunday dinners. But Mom wasn't able to eat them. Despite her insistence on maintaining the tradition, we felt uncomfortable eating in front of her. We realized how much the ritual of sitting down at a table and sharing a meal was tied to our family tradition. Mom eventually progressed to normal food, but we didn't sit at the dining room table and eat as a family until she was able to eat with us.

After a period of working with the home care agency, Mom was hospitalized again. When she returned
home, Mom again required home care. Ironically, the
original home care agency said it could no longer care
for my mom because she was too sick. Although nothing
had changed medically, agency personnel now knew the
Tarantines as the family who asked many questions. Staff
members were used to seeing patients when it was convenient for them, not convenient for the patient. They
weren't used to patients asking questions and wanting to
know why certain things were done. They fired us as
patients.

The need to change home care agencies became a
blessing. I would have never thought that two agencies,
reportedly having the same objective, could provide care
in ways that were so totally different.

The first home care agency was owned by the hospital system in which Mom had been an inpatient. The
second was a faith-based organization, unaffiliated with
any hospital. The new nurse arrived at my house
equipped to assess body, mind, and spirit. The speech
pathologist, Liz, arrived with pages of teaching material.
She said that her job was to teach my mom how to eat
what she wanted and be safe at the same time.

My mother was ecstatic. At last, here was someone
who would allow her to eat what she wanted, with a
tracheostomy in place! Liz told my mother she realized
that eating was important to having a high-quality life.
Liz helped my mother learn what foods were best for her.
Control was given back to Mom, and she knew which
foods she felt safe eating and which foods she didn't.

The physical and occupational therapists changed also. The therapists, Lisa and Jessica, came to assess my

mother. They didn't understand why a 5-foot, 100-pound woman was in a wheelchair designed for a large man. They measured Mom and ordered her a custom wheelchair. They also ordered a special zero-gravity cushion to alleviate the pressure on Mom's bedsore, which was on her coccyx.

The wheelchair cost $3,000 and the cushion cost $1,100. Mom felt like a new woman. She finally had a chair that didn't cause pain at the site of her bedsore. She repeatedly asked me, "How can this be? Why didn't the other agency give me a smaller wheelchair and a special cushion? The hospital caused the bedsore and the home care agency is part of the hospital health system. I just don't understand."

I didn't understand either. The only thing I do understand is this: The hospital system owned the insurance company, the home care agency, and the durable medical equipment (DME) company. After we had an independent and unaffiliated home care agency, equipment was ordered based on my mother's needs rather than what was available at the DME company.

Lisa also arranged to have Susan, a local Eucharistic minister, come to my home every Sunday morning to give my mom Communion. Susan provided the missing link in Mom's care. She added to my mother's quality of life by providing spiritual care. My mother and Susan formed a special relationship over time. Susan even assisted the priest with Communion at my mother's funeral Mass.

* * * * * * *

Throughout my mother's journey, we advocated for her right to live. She believed she had a life of high quality. One day I asked Mom if she would make the same choices again if she knew then what she knew now. "Ruthi, let me tell you something. Your Dad and you kids were my life. I loved being a wife and mother. I am with my children all of the time now. I live with you, and Kath and you take care of me. Bob cares for me every Saturday, and Rick and Debbie care for me on Sunday. We still have Sunday dinner. I have seen Dan and John more in the past two years than I have seen them in the past twenty years. Even Catie takes care of me when she is home from college. What wouldn't I like? I know my life has changed, but when it's your time, it's your time."

That's all I needed to know. Mom's perception was all that mattered in determining the quality of her life. We were fortunate that we knew her wishes prior to her getting sick. She gave us a gift by having a conversation about her wishes with us. We didn't have to guess about what she wanted; we knew. Our job was then to advocate for her, to have her wishes carried out.

A few years back, I had bought my mother a book titled *A Family Legacy for Your Children: Reflections from a Mother's Heart.* The book is a journal; however, it asks specific questions. My mother's last entry was her response to the question "What places would you still like to visit? Why?" This last entry speaks volumes about Mom's life and what she valued, as well as what truly made her happy. Susan, the Eucharistic minister, read this entry at Mom's funeral:

> I have visited a lot of places since I got older. I would like
> to cruise the Mediterranean or see China. However, I am
> at the stage of my life that having my family around me

is the greatest joy I could feel. I feel sorry for the people who are alienated from their families. Life is too short. Enjoy the simple things. You don't have to go anyplace to have happiness.

My mother was neither a diagnosis nor the patient in Room 7, nor the old woman on the ventilator. My mother's Facebook picture was (and still is) a picture of her behind the wheel of my brother's Corvette. We made large 8 by 11 color copies of this picture and hung them in her room. The first one was taped on the door as you walked in. The second one was taped above her head. Our goal was to remind every single person that entered Mom's room that she was a person who had had a life before she came to the hospital. It worked.

Ninety percent of Mom's doctors were men. I've never met a man who didn't like a Corvette. Every person who entered the room commented about that picture. They started to get it: They started to understand why we were advocating for her. She had a life of high quality prior to the hospitalization, and she was determined to resume her life. Maybe Mom's life wouldn't be the same, but it was her choice to keep living. Mom's perception of her quality of life was all that mattered. No one else's.

ACTION STEPS FOR YOUR FAMILY

It has been said that the only thing certain in life is death. It will happen to all of us. We have no choice in the matter. If we are lucky, however, we have a choice in how we die. Whether you are 20 years old or 60 years old, take the time to think about what you would want if you should become seriously ill. Take the initiative to talk about your wishes with your family and friends. Ask them to share their wishes with you.

Do not put off these conversations because they will be uncomfortable discussions or because you think there is plenty of time left. No one knows how much time he or she has left. Give your family members one last gift before you die: Let them know your wishes. It will make a difficult time a bit easier for them. Ask them to give the same gift to you.

1. HOLD CONVERSATIONS AND DOCUMENT YOUR LOVED
    ONES' WISHES
    Talk with your loved ones—parents, siblings, and close relatives, asking them to share their wishes as you share your own. Two documents, a living will and a *Five Wishes* booklet, are available to record a person's wishes. The conversations that surround these documents are hard but essential—insist on them.

2. ENCOURAGE LOVED ONES TO WRITE LIVING WILL
    A living will is a document that can be, but doesn't have to be, written with or by a lawyer. The document should be prepared while the person is well and of sound mind.

    A living will states the person's wishes about end-of-life treatment. It details instructions that medical caregivers should follow in case the person loses the ability to make or communicate decisions. A living will cannot predict every possible treatment choice. Certain choices, however, are common to most end-of-life illnesses, including whether hospital staff should carry out CPR if the heart stops or connect the patient to a breathing machine if the lungs fail.

A living will that states a patient's wish not to be revived if breathing or the heart stops is called a do-not-resuscitate order, or DNR order.

Each state has its own statutes about living wills. Laws vary and may evolve with time, so be sure to update your living will periodically.

It is important to understand that, if a patient does not want to be resuscitated and desires a natural death, a physician must write a DNR order. The terms of the living will are not in effect until the patient or family has a conversation with the doctor, outlining end-of-life wishes, and the doctor writes an order indicating the patient's or family's wishes concerning resuscitation.

3. DOCUMENT FIVE WISHES

The *Five Wishes* booklet is the template for a type of living will that helps a person express how he or she wants to be treated in case of serious illness and inability to communicate. *Five Wishes* is unique among all other living-will and health-agent forms because it provides information about the full scope of a person's needs: medical, personal, emotional, and spiritual. In addition, the content of this document helps structure discussions with family and physicians.

Ask loved ones to specify their five wishes as a gift to family, friends, and their doctor. A document stating wishes keeps others out of the difficult position of having to guess what kind of treatment a patient wants or doesn't want. *Five Wishes* is available from the nonprofit organization Aging with Dignity at http://www.agingwithdignity.org/five-wishes.php.

Five Wishes lets a family and doctors know

- Who the patient wants to make health care decisions when the patient can't make them
- The kind of medical treatment the patient wants or doesn't want
- How comfortable the patient wants to be
- How the patients want people to treat him or her
- What the patient wants loved ones to know

4. SUGGEST APPOINTING A DURABLE POWER OF ATTORNEY

Power of attorney is the ability, legally speaking, to act in someone's place. To be prepared in the case of a loved one becoming mentally incapacitated, ask your loved ones to give someone *durable power of attorney* for medical care and finances. *Durable,* in this case, means that the power of attorney stays in effect from when a person becomes incapacitated until he or she can again handle affairs. Loved ones should appoint someone who knows their wishes and will carry them out. Remember, the person who has durable power of attorney is not to carry out his or her wishes about the end of a person's life, but *that person's* wishes.

5. AS A FAMILY, DISCUSS *QUALITY OF LIFE*

Be careful not to pass judgment on others' definitions. Many things—including our own experiences with death, illness, and suffering—form our wishes concerning our end of life.

My mom wanted everything done to save her life. However, I have siblings who want no intervention if they have cardiac or respiratory failure. Penny, whom I mentioned earlier in this chapter, has a will to live despite not having any limbs. I can also recall Bobby, a patient who chose not to have a cardiac catheterization. He had a family history of heart failure and refused to follow the road of suffering that his father and brothers had. Although many health care providers questioned Bobby's decision and tried to talk him out of refusing the catheterization, he was of sound mind and refused the procedure. Bobby died six months after his refusal.

In acute situations, family members will have a much easier time if they know what their loved one wants and what other loved ones are willing to sacrifice. Some individuals are adamant about going to a nursing home if a time comes for extended care. They have made the choice not to allow other family members to provide needed care. Some families are not able to care for an ill loved one. Each individual's and family's situation is unique. The important thing is that communication occurs among family members—that family members share their wishes.

6. BE PERSISTENT

When your loved one has a quality-of-life issue that health care workers are ignoring or treating as a low priority, persist. You know your loved one and his or her priorities best.

Your persistence is especially important when dealing with specialists, because specialists don't necessarily treat the whole person. Persist until you get any consultation or test you believe is important.

7. CHALLENGE HEALTH CARE PROVIDERS AND INSURANCE
    COMPANIES
    When quality of life is at stake, you don't have to ac-
    cept the answer *That's the way we've always done it.*
    If a procedure is denied, ask why. If you can't get ap-
    proval for the procedure, file an appeal. Don't be
    afraid to escalate the appeal. Individuals who fight to
    change a broken system get results for themselves
    and others.

8. REMEMBER THAT HEALTH CARE PROVIDERS WORK FOR YOU
    If you get the sense that your doctor's ideas about
    end-of-life care will negatively affect your care,
    change doctors. Sometimes a doctor will push a pa-
    tient to continue treatment when the patient would
    rather stop treatment. Sometimes a patient wants
    another round of chemotherapy despite the doctor's
    disagreeing. It is important to have a physician who
    respects your wishes and acknowledges your right to
    choose.

CHAPTER 4

INSIST ON PATIENT-CENTERED CARE

> *The physician should not treat the disease but
> the patient who is suffering from it.*
> ~ Maimonides

O NE EVENING, MY BROTHER, Rick, came straight from
work to the Medical ICU at the trauma center. He
arrived at 7 p.m. and called into the ICU, per their policy,
to request permission to go back and visit Mom. A nurse
said Rick would have to wait until 8:30 p.m. She said they
were giving handoff report, which is a verbal report
about patient care that helps transition care from one
provider to another. In a hospital unit, report occurs at
every shift change.

The nurse explained that it would be a violation of
privacy rules if Rick were in the ICU during report. My
brother offered to go into Mom's room and close the
door. He had just finished his workday and wanted to see
Mom. Rick reminded the nurse that normally Mom was
alone for this hour and a half. He volunteered to leave
the room when the new shift nurse came in to complete
the evening assessment. The nurse answered, "No." Rick
waited thirty minutes and then went in anyway.

By this time, my mother had been in the Medical
ICU for two months. Staff members knew the family

well. They knew we were at the hospital in shifts and were extremely involved in Mom's care. In fact, we made the nurses' jobs easier, since we tended to Mom's needs while there.

We knew how Mom liked her pillow. We knew how many blankets she wanted. We made sure *Jeopardy* was on at 7 p.m., since Mom couldn't work the remote. We rubbed Mom's dry skin with lotion so she wouldn't get another bedsore. We even played cards with her. We did all of the things that made Mom comfortable and feel as though she had some control in her life. To the staff members on duty on this particular night, none of this mattered. The rules were the rules.

When Rick walked into the ICU, the nurse immediately told him he would have to leave. Rick asked her why. The nurse cited privacy rules and again Rick said he would shut the door. Rick said, "I've been waiting and watching through the tiny window in the ICU doors. I've been watching the staff nurses talking and laughing while my mother is alone in her room. You are obviously done with report.

"While you are sitting here talking, the waiting room is full of upset family members. We are tired after working all day and want to see our loved ones. Visiting hours are over at 9 p.m. If we wait until 8:30 as you are insisting, that will leave us with only thirty minutes of visiting time. Besides, my mother is much more relaxed when family members are in her room. She becomes anxious when she knows we are in the waiting room and aren't allowed to come in."

The nurse growled in response, "This has always been our rule. Families are not permitted into the ICU until 8:30." After a moment she snapped, "Fine. Go in and close the door."

This has always been our rule. This sentence captures a recurring theme throughout my mother's illness. Mom came to the hospital a mentally sharp and independent woman. After she arrived, she was expected to give up control. Mom's care was based on the needs and values of those who provided care rather than customized to match her needs and values. Each nurse and physician had different needs and values, so Mom's care was always subject to their personal perspectives. She was subject to provider-centered care rather than patient-centered care. The only needs and values that should have mattered were those of my mother, the patient.

Obviously, it is sometimes inappropriate to have families in the ICU or other acute care areas. The presence of families is not always compatible with maintaining patients' privacy and dignity. Many people, including other families, can unwittingly violate a patient's privacy. Whole families often walk down a hall and glare into every room before getting to their loved one's room. Nonetheless, this behavior doesn't justify the arbitrary *no visitors during report* policy and others that are provider-centered rather than patient-centered.

Fortunately, a shift is occurring in health care, albeit at an excruciatingly slow pace. With many studies showing that U.S. health care is subpar, governing bodies are pushing hospitals to patient-centered care, by using financial incentives. Hospital administrators across the country are beginning to realize that involving families in care will help them provide safer, less expensive care.

For example, patients fall frequently in hospitals across the country. These falls cost millions in lawsuits as well as increased lengths of stay. It just makes sense to encourage families to be in patient rooms as often as possible. A few hospitals currently encourage families to spend the night, even in acute care settings. These hospitals provide family members with a comfortable cot, bedding, and an attitude that conveys, "We want your loved one to be safe and receive the best possible care—and you can help. Let's be partners."

As a nurse, I have experienced the patient-centered approach firsthand and seen it make a world of difference. For a time, I was employed as a contract agency nurse (traveling nurse), working at hospitals across the country. Also, I spent time in Palermo, Italy, assisting in opening a new transplant hospital.

My first traveling contract was in sunny Hawaii, where I cared for Samuk, a large 40-year-old Samoan man who was unconscious because of a recent stroke. Hawaii is a melting pot of many cultures, and hospitals are used to accommodating the individual needs of patients. In fact, my brief hospital orientation there focused on the etiquette of caring for patients from various cultures.

I recall walking into Samuk's room to begin the night shift, at 7 p.m., and being overwhelmed. I counted 14 family members in the small room. I was overcome with the aroma of kalua pig. The family was having dinner, and I was unable to make my way to the patient through the crowded room. I remember asking for permission to assess their loved one. This was new for me, having last worked at a transplant unit in a large trauma center. The family willingly made a path for me.

As I reached the bedside, I saw that the unresponsive patient was covered in large green leaves. I was stunned. My mind went a mile a minute. "What about infection? Did anyone wash these leaves? What if there is an emergency? The Code Team can't even get into the room. Don't they know this is a hospital?" I thought.

Noticing my expression, a family member answered my unspoken concerns. "These are special tea leaves," she said. "Samoans have used these for hundreds of years to cure disease. We thought it couldn't hurt," continued the patient's sister, Suki. "When you get time, can you bring us a couple of recliners so we can spend the night? Most of us will be leaving, but my mother and I want to spend the night with Samuk."

The Hawaiian hospital had an abundance of recliners specifically for families. Working around the recliners that night, I realized that Samuk's family could provide a type of care I never could. They anticipated what Samuk might need because they knew him.

I also experienced patient-centered care at a Native American hospital in Alaska. Assessing the use of herbal remedies and respecting tribal traditions was integral in customizing patient care. In fact, a non-native nurse was not trusted until the patient saw evidence that the nurse respected his or her culture and values.

As part of a team of providers from a transplant unit, I traveled to Palermo, Italy, to help open a transplant hospital. Although transplant center staff members attempted to educate us about cultural differences, they couldn't begin to prepare us for our interactions with patients' families, Italian doctors, and the Italian nun who ran the nursing unit.

Families visited at their convenience, not ours. Italian doctors treated patients and families with respect, and the respect was reciprocated. Family members brought pasta from home for patients. Patients commonly had wine with their dinners.

I recall walking into a patient's room a few days after the patient had undergone a liver transplant. The patient was eating pasta with marinara sauce and sausage. I was aghast: The typical plan of care called for a clear liquid diet. When I asked who gave the patient the pasta, the head nurse, an Italian nun, responded in broken English, "I did. The only way for patient to get better is to *mangi, mangi.*"

The patient did get better. So much for the clear liquid diet. So much for no wine with dinner. Despite the standards of care and rules the Americans brought to Italy, with the intent to teach Italians how to deliver quality care to transplant patients, the Americans were the ones who walked away with an enhanced understanding of how culture and values support recovery. I never forgot the lessons I learned there.

THE DRIVE TOWARD PATIENT-CENTERED CARE IN THE UNITED STATES

Although the United States has unrivaled status in many areas, health care is not one of them. As mentioned earlier, the World Health Organization ranked the United States 37th in health care quality in the world in 2000 (Murray & Frenk, 2010). In 2004, 2006, 2007, and 2010, the Commonwealth Fund, an organization that conducts independent research and provides grants to improve health care practice and policies, completed more studies.

These studies, reported by Davis, Schoen, and Stremikis (2010), compared U.S. health system performance to that in six other industrialized countries: Australia, Canada, Germany, the Netherlands, New Zealand, and the United Kingdom. Performance was measured in terms of quality; efficiency; access to care; equity; and the ability to lead a long, healthy, productive life.

Despite spending the most money on health care, the United States ranks dead last. The most significant way the United States differs from other countries is in the absence of universal health care coverage. But even when access and equity measures are not considered, the United States is behind most of the other countries on most measures.

As a result, American governing bodies are insisting that hospitals improve care by moving toward patient-centered care and by taking other quality-improvement measures. The surveys you receive after visiting a doctor or medical facility are designed to measure patient satisfaction and the level of patient-centered care. Medical provider reimbursement will be increasingly based on the scores from such surveys. Accordingly, everyone in health care is talking about patient-centered care.

Here's a simple definition of *patient-centered care:* Nothing about me without me (Delbanco et al., 2001). However, the landmark book *Crossing the Quality Chasm: A New Healthcare System for the 21st Century* (CQHCA, 2001), published by the Institute of Medicine (IOM), makes the definition more complicated. This report defines patient-centered care as "care that is respectful of and responsive to individual patient preferences, needs, and values and [ensures] that patient values guide all clinical decisions."

According to the IOM report, patient-centeredness is one of six aims for quality improvement in health care. The others are safety, timeliness, effectiveness, efficiency, and equity.

Realizing that health care cannot change overnight, the IOM offered 10 simple rules to redesign health care (CQHCA, 2001). A link in the References section (at the end of the book) leads to an online summary of the IOM rules. The rules appear to be based on common sense, but individuals who have been in a hospital recently know that patient control is still an issue in U.S. hospitals. Typically, a patient gives up control the moment he or she walks in the door. We Americans accept this as normal because it has been the standard for so long.

Although foreign to long-standing practice in U.S. health care, research shows that patient-centered care yields better results.

- Patients who participate in their care have better outcomes overall.
- Patients are more likely to follow a plan of care when they help to design the plan.
- Patients who receive patient-centered care report higher patient-satisfaction scores.

Unfortunately, for most patients, patient-centered care is an anomaly.

Hospitals are rapidly trying to change their culture to one of patient-centered care. Even so, hospitals often miss the mark. A great deal of money is being spent on educating hospital staff on the definition of *patient-centered care.* The problem, however, isn't lack of understanding of the definition. The problem is putting patient-centered care into practice. The culture of control is so engrained in U.S. health care that a major shift in thinking is needed.

Patient-centered care requires dynamic human interaction between patient (and the patient's advocates) and health care providers. Each patient will have different input because each patient is unique. It is a provider's job to integrate the patient's input into the plan to achieve optimal results.

You might think of patient-centered care as going back to the Golden Rule of treating others the way you want to be treated. Unfortunately, the way you want to be treated isn't necessarily the way someone else wants to be treated. Care that assumes the provider knows what the patient wants is still provider-centered. Patient-centered care requires providers to ask the patient or family what the patient prefers.

Patient-centered care thrives when patients and/or their advocates play two roles: partner and source of feedback.

In patient-centered care, the patient or the patient's advocate functions as a partner, working in collaboration with the physician and staff. The patient or advocate collaborates with the health care provider to make decisions and help manage the patient's care. Collaboration with a physician helps that physician care for the patient according to the patient's needs, values, and priorities. Active participation in a partnership role is crucial for a successful outcome.

In addition to acting as health care partners, patients and/or advocates are a source of essential feedback to the medical team. The patient's perspective provides unique feedback to the provider, helping gauge the effectiveness of care, as well as the performance of the provider or organization. Surveys of patients provide helpful feedback after the fact, but no one should wait for a survey to communicate.

Providers naturally look at things through the lens of a physician or nurse rather than the lens of the patient. If you are unhappy with your care or see an opportunity to improve it, speak up. This is your obligation. Providers can't make a course correction after the fact. They can't fix a problem until they know they have one. Your participation in providing feedback is crucial for a successful outcome.

In many cases, you won't get patient-centered care unless you relentlessly pursue it. With perseverance, however, you can get exceptions to hospital and insurance practices to customize your loved one's care and improve his or her quality of life. Be present. Ask questions. Speak up. Keep good records. Learn to think beyond *how it is always done* and to speak in dollars and cents. Refuse to be intimidated. Most important, don't give up.

Perseverance helped our family achieve multiple successes in getting approval for treatments or practices outside the norm. One of these attracted spectators in the ICU.

An ICU patient's anxiety is often a barrier to weaning the patient from a ventilator. The patient is afraid of not being able to breathe while being weaned. Unfortunately, elderly patients, including my mother, have few medication options when it comes to decreasing anxiety.

Decreasing my mother's anxiety was crucial as we tried to ready her for discharge. As Mom's advocate, I decided to ask her ICU physician, Dr. Daniels, to try something different, something that perhaps only Mom and my family would be willing to try. I wanted Dr. Daniels to approve a patient-centered treatment for Mom's anxiety.

The trauma center's health system included a department of integrative medicine. The department offered acupuncture. I asked Dr. Daniels if I could have an acupuncturist assess my mother, to see if treatments could help with anxiety. He agreed. Whether this was because Dr. Daniels was patient-centered or simply eager to do anything that would help my mother wean from the ventilator, and ultimately discharge her and our pesky family from his ICU, we will never know.

Dr. Daniels wrote the order for acupuncture, which allowed L. L. Wei, licensed acupuncturist, to treat my mom. Although skeptical of having needles inserted into her body, Mom agreed, saying, "What do I have to lose at this point?"

As the acupuncturist was treating Mom, a cluster of health care workers looked in. Amazed, Mom asked, "What are they looking at? There must be ten doctors and nurses looking in here. Don't they know I can see them?"

"Well, they've never seen someone getting acupuncture before, let alone in the ICU," I said. "It's not every day staff members see a patient with needles sticking out of her forehead, ears, and neck."

In Mom's ears, L. L. Wei left needles with little magnets on the ends. He taught family members how to attach small magnets to the end of the magnets on the needles in her ears. We were to turn them back and forth six times a day for a total of six days. We were all out of our comfort zone. It didn't matter. This is what my mother and family members were willing to try to help alleviate anxiety related to ventilator weaning.

The acupuncture treatment for anxiety was a first for the ICU and clinicians, something that would never have occurred without a specific request from a patient's advocate. I can't say definitively whether the treatment worked or not, but I do know that my mother's time on the vent became increasingly less over the next few weeks. Her anxiety appeared to be under control.

PARTNERING WITH LIKE-MINDED THINKERS

In any organization, there will be individuals who tend to think alike. Oftentimes, these individuals gravitate toward one another. People who are known to think out of the box tend to know like-minded thinkers.

Finding doctors or nurses willing to advocate for a loved one and try something new isn't always easy. We were lucky to find a few providers who went the extra mile for my mom and ultimately changed the course of her journey. The following stories provide some insight into how to identify such individuals. More important, the stories illustrate the way in which such individuals are connected to other advocates who can assist on the journey to patient-centered care.

A few days after the ICU-visiting issue with Rick, Kathy came to the ICU at the trauma center around 10 a.m. Typically, each morning Mom was helped out of bed and taken off the ventilator for a few hours. The goal was to advance the length of time off the ventilator each day until Mom could be off it entirely.

On this particular day, Kathy arrived to find my mother in bed, receiving her dialysis treatment. Kathy asked the nurse if my mother had been out of bed and off the ventilator that morning. The nurse said Mom had not been out of bed, because of dialysis.

Kathy thought this was odd. She asked the nurse why they had performed dialysis in the morning rather than the evening. The nurse said, "This is the way they always do dialysis."

Kathy asked for the telephone number of the Dialysis Unit. She spoke to the charge nurse, who was quick to point out that the department performs dialysis on many patients in three adjoining hospitals. They can't take requests.

Kathy explained that she was merely asking for dialysis to be performed after 3 p.m. This would allow my mother to get out of bed and wean from the ventilator. As things stood, my mother's recovery was slowed because of her dialysis schedule. The charge nurse insisted that this could not be done. "After all," she stated, "We are a Level I trauma center with a lot of sick ICU patients."

Kathy became frustrated. It just made sense to dialyze our mother in the afternoon. Kathy couldn't understand why no one else saw this as obvious. "Don't they realize that the longer Mom stays here, the more money it costs the hospital? The more potential there is for another infection? For another bedsore? Mom needs to be weaned from the vent to leave the ICU. Why isn't this a priority?" she questioned.

Kathy asked to talk to the nurse manager in the Dialysis Unit, Mary, and repeated the story. Mary responded, "It makes perfect sense to me. Sure, we can do that. I will schedule your Mom to be dialyzed on the second shift, 3 to 11 p.m. I can't schedule a specific time, but your mom's dialysis will be after 3 p.m.," she stated matter-of-factly.

It took conversations with three nurses before achieving a patient-centered dialysis schedule. It took three conversations before someone listened and thought about Kathy's request. A simple fix changed a practice that was delaying my mother's recovery and transfer out of the ICU.

What's more, that simple change saved the hospital money. Although my mother had a Medicare Advantage Plan through a private insurance company, the insurance company was owned by the hospital's health system. My mother's length of stay directly affected the health system financially. After a patient exceeds the average length of stay for a diagnosis, the hospital begins to lose money on that patient, unless hospital staff can provide medical justification for the extension of stay. Decisions affecting length of stay are fiscal as well as medical.

Kathy persisted until she found a person with decision-making power who could think outside the box. Mary listened to Kathy's request and actually thought about what she was asking. Rather than making Kathy feel as though Kathy was a pain by askng for a change in the normal routine, Mary saw the request as an opportunity to improve the care the hospital was giving my mother. Mary's attitude toward patient-centered care made all the difference.

We didn't know it at the time, but Mary would play a crucial role in my mother's recovery and quality of life for the rest of Mom's days. A few months after Mary honored Kathy's request for a schedule change, Mom's doctor informed us that he would allow us to take Mom home with the ventilator. The tracheostomy, however, continued to be a barrier to outpatient dialysis.

Again, Mary came to our rescue. We didn't know Mary. She had never seen my mother—Mary was usually in the Dialysis Unit, running the show, not in the ICU, dialyzing patients. Mary knew only that my mother was a patient who had a trach, wanted to go home, and needed dialysis. Period. Mary agreed to dialyze my mother in her unit, as an outpatient. Because of Mary's willingness to customize care for a patient, my mother was able to go home. Although Mary's Dialysis Unit was an inpatient facility, the unit also had an outpatient license, so she agreed to dialyze Mom as an outpatient.

People like Mary, who have patient-centered care engrained in their souls, tend to associate with others with the same philosophy. Mary's unit consisted of a pocket of nurses and physicians who were used to placing the patient at the center of care. We accompanied my mother, via ambulance, three times a week to the Dialysis Unit under Mary's supervision. There, Mom received care I haven't witnessed anyplace in my twenty-five years of nursing. My mother was in control from the moment she entered the unit. Information flowed freely, and it became a patient-provider partnership based on trust, respect, and collaboration.

At one point, my mother acquired a dialysis-catheter infection whose treatment required an expensive and potent IV antibiotic. The insurance company advised us that the co-pay would be $150 per dose. This potent antibiotic was not normally given in an outpatient dialysis setting, so this was uncharted territory for the insurance company. Mom was an outlier.

My mother needed to have the antibiotic infused after 14 dialysis treatments, which equated to a period of almost five weeks. The insurance company declared that Mom had to go to a nursing home for the infusions. Once again, Mary intervened by contacting the insurance company. She reminded the company that waiving the co-pay would cost much less than paying for a five-week stay in a nursing facility. Mary offered to administer the drug in her unit after every dialysis treatment.

Dollars and cents became a recurring theme in my mom's illness. We found that, when our case was presented in dollars and cents, the likelihood of the request being granted rose exponentially. Sure, providers and insurers had guidelines for disease management, but once challenged with the economics of a decision, they would usually change their minds. We learned.

Our goal became to find that person who could add 2 plus 2 and who had the power to make decisions. Finding that person was tough at times, but perseverance paid off. It wasn't easy to recite the same story repeatedly. In fact, it is easy to see why a family member might just give up. However, there is no greater reward than knowing you are forging the way for change and helping your loved one—not to mention future patients and families. There really are many compassionate people out there who will help you.

We continued to find compassionate people along the way. My family and I realized my mother would most likely be spending the rest of her life making trips three times a week to the trauma center for dialysis. Transportation took about three hours round trip, coupled with a four-hour dialysis treatment. While we were grateful to be accepted for outpatient dialysis, I felt there had to be a better way.

Mary and I spoke about the possibility of home dialysis. Home hemodialysis, while once rare, is now becoming commonplace. Outpatient centers usually have a home dialysis arm and nurses who train the patient and family how to dialyze at home. The issue for us, however, was that outpatient centers can't accept anyone with a tracheostomy, so this automatically excluded my mother from the possibility of home dialysis. That is, until Mary reached out to her colleagues at an area outpatient dialysis center.

Initially, the outpatient dialysis center refused to accept my mother for the home dialysis program, because of the tracheostomy. Center managers were just following the rules. Again, we had to look for a like-minded thinker who dared to break away from the *we've always done it this way* mentality.

In this case, the person was Dr. Belista, who, as medical director of the outpatient dialysis center, agreed to take my mother as a patient in the Home Dialysis Program. Dr. Belista went out on a limb, and it paid off for my mother and my family. No more trips to the trauma center for dialysis. Instead, my mother was dialyzed on my sun porch, watching the deer and birds feed. My mother went from having to sleep after her traditional four-hour treatment to doing physical therapy after her two-hour home treatments.

Things still weren't necessarily easy. Since my mother had a tracheostomy, the outpatient center was not permitted to be the much-needed dialysis backup in case something went wrong. Once again, Mary came to the rescue: She agreed to make her center our backup. In October 2011, my mother became the first person with a tracheostomy to receive home hemodialysis in the state of Pennsylvania.

Home hemodialysis drastically improved my mother's quality of life. It saved travel time while allowing Mom to be in a comfortable environment. Although it may seem that our family went to the extreme in learning how to dialyze at home, that's not necessarily true. Most caregivers who perform home hemodialysis have absolutely no health care experience. In fact, the patient and family member that the outpatient center trained prior to my mom and me were a 70-year-old married couple with no background in health care.

For our family, the biggest barrier wasn't learning how to dialyze, it was finding a way to measure Mom's fluid retention. We needed a wheelchair scale, which cost around $1,000. It seemed there had to be a cheaper way. And there was. I found a llama scale on the Internet for $299. The scale was brand-new and perfect for rolling a wheelchair onto. It was digital and accurate. My mother fondly referred to herself as Mama Llama.

My mother received hemodialysis at home for almost a year before she died. She visited the dialysis clinic monthly, per Medicare guidelines, to have blood drawn and receive new supplies. She saw a dietitian and social worker in addition to a physician and nurse. Mom filled out a quality-of-life survey monthly and rated her quality of life as a 9 out of 10, with 10 being the highest. Mom often joked that she would have rated her life a 10 if it hadn't been for the monthly visits to the center for lab work and supplies.

NAVIGATING THE WORLD OF NONHOSPITAL INSTITUTIONS

Hospitals weren't the only places at which we had to struggle to receive patient-centered care. We faced the frustrating motto *the way we always do things* in regard to equipment and supplies, too. Once again, persistence paid off.

Although we received some of our supplies from the dialysis center, the rest were delivered via various insurance-approved vendors. My sister and I ordered all supplies monthly, dealing with multiple vendors to get what my mother needed. I can recall the weeks following my mother's initial hospital discharge. The company that provided all the DME was owned by the hospital's health system. We were allotted a specific number of supplies per Medicare guidelines. No one took into account my mother's condition, past medical history, or current needs. The only thing that mattered was adherence to Medicare guidelines.

Despite the fact that my mother suffered from recurring pneumonia, first acquired in the hospital, the DME company allotted only so many suction catheters per month. We were expected to wash the catheters in a vinegar solution and reuse them. These catheters were going through the opening in Mom's neck and trachea and down into her lungs to retrieve secretions.

Although the average home is much cleaner than a hospital, allowing an infection-control regimen less rigorous than a hospital's, reusing catheters still didn't make sense. Our goal was to keep the pneumonia at bay and thereby avoid a hospital readmission. Again, I wondered, "Isn't there someone who realizes that a hospital admission costs more than the $2 catheters?"

My family members were washing suction catheters, gastric containers and tubing, and other equipment that required disassembly and then reassembly, all the while hoping we would reassemble the items correctly. We were spending more time washing supplies than providing direct care. Something had to give.

After multiple discussions with Don, the man in the warehouse at the DME company, we were informed that, if a doctor's prescription indicated that we needed more than the Medicare allotment of catheters, the company would supply them. I informed Dr. Daniels, the pulmonologist who initially discharged my mother from the hospital, of the need for more catheters. He immediately took out his prescription pad and wrote an order to suction my mother every two hours and as needed, with a new catheter. I faxed the order to the DME company. Within twenty-four hours, we had 240 catheters. Once again, with persistence, we found an answer, another simple fix to achieve patient-centered rather than provider-centered care.

ACTION STEPS FOR YOUR FAMILY

1. INSIST ON PATIENT-CENTERED CARE
    Signing the Consent to Treat form upon admission to the hospital is not synonymous with writing, "I give all control to you to do whatever you please to my body."

    You have the right to demand patient-centered care for yourself or your loved one. Accept nothing less. If your physician doesn't embrace patient-centered care, change doctors. If your nurse refuses to include you in your own plan of care, ask for a different nurse. If you find this difficult, remind yourself that your goal in health care is not to make friends, but to get the optimal outcome. For optimal outcomes, patients, families, and providers all need to be on the same page.

Remember: Nothing about me without me. The patient has the right to ultimate control in the hospital, and providers should not take control without permission from the patient.

2. ASK QUESTIONS AND MAKE REQUESTS AS A COLLABORATOR
    Transparency and information sharing are crucial ingredients in patient-centered care. You have the right and responsibility to understand your own or your loved one's plan of care. At the same time, take care to present your questions and requests as a collaborator rather than an adversary.

    Ask for printed material on a diagnosis or procedure. Ask for printed information on medications. Ask your providers to recommend websites that provide helpful or supplemental information. Information should flow freely to patients and families.

    If you have questions about why one treatment is chosen over another, ask. If you believe some alternative treatment would benefit your loved one, discuss it.

3. ACCEPT RESPONSIBILITY TO PROVIDE FEEDBACK
    Patient-centered care is a two-way street. Let your doctor, nurse, or hospital administrator know when you are unhappy or a plan of care is not working. You might have an unpleasant conversation with a few people before you get results, but at the end of

the day, it will be worth it. Hospitals, doctors, and nurses need to know they are doing the wrong thing in order to fix it.

It might be easy to walk away and internalize your frustration with a broken system, but this will quickly wear on you and your family. Speak up!

4. PERSIST IN LOOKING FOR PROVIDERS WHO THINK IN TERMS OF PATIENT-CENTERED CARE

Be relentless in looking for those pockets of providers who provide patient-centered care. Find those passionate providers who think outside the box. Many of these individuals can move mountains to get things done. Acknowledge those who go out of their way to help you.

Remember that like-minded people tend to attract each other. Sometimes, it is beneficial to mention a barrier you are encountering to a provider who has helped you in the past. Many times, that provider knows someone who can help or can at least point you in the right direction to accomplish your goal. Communicating your needs is crucial to finding those who will help you.

5. LEARN TO SPEAK IN DOLLARS AND CENTS

Money talks, whether you are dealing with the hospital, Medicare, Medicaid, DME company, or insurance company. Before you go to bat for yourself or a loved one, write down your thoughts. On the Internet, do a little homework on how much things cost.

Prepare your points before beginning a telephone conversation or meeting. Be the first to bring up dollars and cents. Providers won't initiate such a conversation because they don't want to appear to be focused on money only. However, everyone has to answer to someone about money being spent. The case manager must answer to the boss when a patient is not discharged in a timely fashion. The DME employee must answer to the boss when he or she sends the patient more catheters than allowed.

One of the biggest failures of our nation's health care system is the inability to understand fully the meaning of *penny-wise and pound-foolish*. Remind providers that saving a few dollars only to have a patient readmitted with an infection is counterproductive. Insist on a long-term rather than a short-term financial perspective.

CHAPTER 5

NAVIGATE A BROKEN HEALTH CARE SYSTEM

> *Accept—then act. Whatever the present moment contains, accept it as if you had chosen it. Always work with it, not against it. Make it your friend and ally, not your enemy. This will miraculously transform your whole life.*
>
> ~ Eckhart Tolle

THE TELEPHONE CALL CAME on Monday, without warning, just one week into my mother's initial hospitalization in the ICU at the community hospital.

"Hi, Ruth. This is Beth, the wound care nurse from the hospital. I'm sorry to call you, but I was told to let you know your mom has a pressure ulcer, a bedsore. When I saw her last Tuesday, the skin on her tailbone was red. I classified it as a stage I pressure ulcer and entered recommendations for care into the computer. The doctor should have seen my recommendations, but I guess something happened with the computerized charting. I came back to work today, after the weekend, and saw your mom. The wound is now at stage III. Your mom has an open wound with full-thickness tissue loss. I don't know how this happened."

"You have to be kidding," I responded. "How did my mother go from a red area on her tailbone to an open wound that severe in five days? Wasn't anyone looking at her skin? I know the nurses are required to assess her skin every four hours at a minimum, per hospital policy. Why didn't you or the other wound care nurse see my mom on Wednesday through Friday, after you identified the stage I sore on her tailbone? I just don't understand."

"I wrote recommendations in the e-record. For some reason the doctor didn't see them. I don't know what to say. The administrators are investigating to see what happened," Beth whispered as she hung up the phone.

I tried to understand what had happened. As an ICU patient, my mom was at high risk for a bedsore, and staff members knew that. Everyone in the ICU is at high risk for a bedsore. Assessing a patient's skin is paramount, since ICU patients can't usually reposition their bodies by themselves. A bedsore this severe should never happen. I knew it, and hospital staff knew it. My mother was the victim of a never event. I headed to the hospital for answers.

As I walked into the ICU, you could hear a pin drop. Staff members knew I had been notified of the wound. I entered Mom's room while her nurse, Jodi, was administering Mom's meds. "I guess you heard," Jodi said matter-of-factly.

"I did hear, and I need to know why this happened. I also need to know what the plan of care is now."

Jodi reviewed the plan of care and said the ICU team of doctors and nurses were still trying to figure out what had happened. "I am so sorry, but it happens," she stated, as if what had happened were an everyday occurrence.

I sat in Mom's room for over two hours before the unit director, Juliana, came in. She put on a gown and gloves before sitting down. I asked Juliana why she had *gowned up.*

"Your mom has a VRE. We culture everyone in the ICU, and she came back positive." Juliana was referring to an infection with vancomycin-resistant enterococci, VRE, a very difficult-to-treat infection. "Your mother picked it up somewhere," Juliana said calmly.

"My mom didn't have an infection when they cultured her on admission. So she now has a hospital-acquired infection and developed a bedsore, all in one week?" I said in disbelief. "She had one problem at admission and now has three serious problems after one week in your care."

"I'm sorry, but it happens sometimes, Ruth. You know that. I am meeting with the director of nursing this afternoon, so we can figure out why this happened. I'll let you know what we find out," she said, while removing her gown and gloves.

I was appalled. A nurse had noticed Mom's red skin last Tuesday. Even if the e-record failed on some level, many nurses had cared for Mom since Tuesday. They should have caught the problem. In addition, my mother now had VRE, an infection typically transmitted by health care workers who did not wash their hands between patient contact.

This is the exact point at which the transition occurred for me. During my mom's third week in her first hospitalization, I psychologically and emotionally went from the nurse and employee of a hospital to the daughter and advocate my mother needed. I couldn't straddle the line between the two. Nothing else mattered as I gathered the strength I would need to navigate a broken and inept health care system.

Juliana had summed up the problem succinctly, "I'm sorry, but it happens sometimes." No matter how compassionate and competent the doctors and nurses and no matter the health care facility, health care workers function within a broken system, where communication and coordination of care break down on a regular basis. Patients need family members to be vigilant on their behalf.

By the time my Mom was transferred from the community hospital to the LTAC facility, a few months later, Mom's bedsore had become a stage IV wound. When a bedsore arrives at stage III, it is extremely difficult to stop the progression to stage IV.

The bedsore affected every aspect of Mom's recovery. The associated pain was so intense that frequent doses of IV narcotics stopped helping. Although her wound improved over time, a stage IV wound can never revert to a prior stage. Stage IV bedsores are deep, with exposed bone, tendons, or muscle. The threat of a bone infection is always looming.

The high doses of narcotics and unrelieved pain of the bedsore increased the difficulty of weaning from the ventilator. It was painful for Mom to sit in a chair and expand her lungs, because the wound was on her tailbone.

Months after the onset of the bedsore, when we were caring for Mom at home, Mom continued to see a plastic surgeon, Dr. Blackwell, as an outpatient for wound care. Dr. Blackwell was the wound doctor who had cared for my mother at the LTAC facility. Despite his training as a surgeon, Dr. Blackwell's specialty is the medical management of wounds. This is rare, since surgeons typically look to surgery for solutions. Dr. Blackwell recommends surgery only after all else fails.

Dr. Blackwell began to wonder why Mom's bedsore wasn't getting smaller, despite his treatment. Beginning to worry that Mom had a bone infection, Dr. Blackwell ordered a CT scan of her tailbone area. He called me with the report. "The radiologist said the CT is consistent with the CT they did three months ago at the hospital. It shows advanced osteomyelitis—bone infection. Did you know about this?" he questioned.

"*No!*" I burst out. "I knew nothing about this. Are you telling me the hospital had this information three months ago and no one noticed?"

I learned that Dr. Farrell knew nothing about the bone infection. Apparently, when the hospital had performed a CT scan a few months earlier, on Mom's groin area, no one had bothered to finish reading the whole report, which indicated that Mom had a bone infection. I was outraged. In addition, I learned a lesson I would never forget. From that moment forward, I requested a copy of every test result. As ridiculous as it seemed, the job of care coordination and communication was in the lap of our family.

We learned that the chronic infection wouldn't kill my mother; it would just advance and cause her more pain. Dr. Blackwell recommended that Mom continue with medical management of the wound, such as dressing changes with an antibiotic cream. He prescribed a topical pain medication that gave Mom some relief.

Although Dr. Blackwell helped Mom receive some pain relief, she began to see a pain specialist at a hospital pain clinic. The pain doctor reviewed Mom's chart, which cited numerous iatrogenic events. The doctor vowed she would ensure that something like that wouldn't happen at her clinic. Little did the well-intended doctor know that she would add to the string of iatrogenic events. She prescribed a new pain medication, which Mom took as prescribed, but the dosage was too high for a renal patient. The result was an overdose and emergency dialysis for my mother.

After this incident, Mom stopped looking for new ways to control her pain and learned to live with it. This required high doses of narcotics that were mostly ineffective. Although the bedsore would slowly improve and become smaller, the infection and pain never went away. Mom went to her grave with that bedsore, 2½ years after acquiring it.

After the pain medication overdose, our family insisted that all new drug prescriptions and all changes in medication doses be made only with the approval of the nephrologist, Mom's kidney doctor. Other doctors weren't pleased with this, but once again, our family had learned to monitor communication and coordination of care.

Unbelievably, these are just snippets of adverse events that Mom experienced in the hospital. Some nights, I reread over and over the Eckhart Tolle quote that begins this chapter. I stopped responding with shock to mistakes and adverse events. I started to expect health care to be broken and embrace my role as advocate within that system. After I accepted the state of affairs in health care, everything became easier. To think that I could change the process and system was foolish. All I needed to change was the care that my mother received.

I learned to embrace this flawed system as though I had chosen it. I made changes in my mother's care regimen based on what I knew was working. I tried to safeguard against mistakes, such as by acquiring a copy of the results of every test and having the kidney doctor authorize all changes in Mom's medications. I learned to work within the tangled maze of health care, always assuming that processes would fail. Being proactive versus reactive in care coordination helped us avoid even more mistakes and adverse effects.

OFFICIAL ATTEMPTS AT SAFEGUARDING OUR HEALTH CARE SYSTEM

On the best of days, health care can be organized chaos. On the worst of days, health care is a dysfunctional hodgepodge of reactive individuals. Although it may provide little solace when your loved one's life is at stake, official organizations and accrediting bodies are trying not only to improve patient safety, but also to guide hospitals to do the same. Organizations such as the National Quality Forum (NQF) and Joint Commission are integral to providing guidance to hospitals.

In a perfect world, hospitals would develop safety initiatives based on identified gaps in care, with the aim of improving overall quality. In the real world, money plays an important part in those initiatives. Therefore, it becomes necessary for outside organizations to mandate that hospitals meet safety guidelines to obtain accreditation.

The Joint Commission, an independent not-for-profit organization, evaluates and accredits more than 20,000 health care organizations and programs in the United

States. The goal of the Joint Commission (2013a) is to "improve health care for the public, in collaboration with other stakeholders, by evaluating health care organizations and inspiring them to excel in providing safe and effective care of the highest quality and value."

Since 1995, the commission has recommended that hospitals report all *sentinel events* to the Joint Commission. A sentinel event is defined as "an unexpected occurrence involving death or serious physiological or psychological injury, or the risk thereof" (Joint Commission, 2008).

Never events, as defined by the NQF, are also considered sentinel events by the commission. The commission mandates performance of a root-cause analysis after any sentinel event.

The Leapfrog Group, representing patient safety and many of the nation's largest corporations and public agencies that buy health benefits, recommends more than a root-cause analysis. The group recommends that health care organizations disclose the error that causes a sentinel event, apologize to the patient, report the event, and waive all costs associated with the event.

Never events, like my mom's bedsore, are devastating and preventable. Health care organizations are capable of eliminating them completely if they have an incentive. Although the delivery of quality care should be the incentive, this hasn't historically been the case. The catalyst for quick change has always been money.

Finally, the Centers for Medicare & Medicaid Services announced in August 2007 that Medicare would no longer pay for the costs associated with many preventable errors, including those considered never events. Since then, many states and private insurers have adopted similar policies.

NATIONAL PATIENT-SAFETY GOALS

In addition to a list of never events, the Joint Commission has a list of national patient-safety goals. Patients and advocates who familiarize themselves with safety goals are in a position to insist providers reach them. The list, begun by the Joint Commission in 2003, is based on identified areas of concern for safety. Most of the goals were added after analysis showed that many reported errors related to a specific area.

For example, it became clear that many errors were related to patient identification. As a result, the Joint Commission mandated that two patient identifiers, such as name and birthdate or medical record number, be verified before medication is given or a procedure or test is performed. Obviously, quality care begins with ensuring you are treating the correct patient.

Here are the Joint Commission (2013b) national patient-safety goals for hospitals:

- Identify patients correctly.
- Use medicines safely.
- Improve staff communication.
- Prevent infection.
- Identify patient-safety risks.
- Prevent mistakes in surgery.

Many subcategories appear under each goal. In addition, there are different safety goals for different types of facilities, such as facilities that provide home care, behavioral health care, and long-term care, to name a few.

WORKING WITH INDIVIDUALS PROVIDING HEALTH CARE

As families navigate through the broken health care system, they will have short- and long-term interactions with doctors, nurses, therapists, technicians, administrators, insurance professionals, and more. Unfortunately, a person in any one of these categories may be a bully, a person as broken as the system within which he or she works. Although only a small percentage of providers fall into this category, families need to be ready to address bully behavior that may compromise a loved one's care.

My mother and family encountered only one bully provider, although that one was more than enough. Dr. Silvers was the surgeon who operated on Mom for the gastrointestinal problems she experienced shortly after her first admission to the community hospital. Dr. Silvers' bully behavior rippled throughout the team that cared for my mother, necessitating my family to demand the care, communication, and respect Mom deserved.

For example, I remember Dr. Silvers' resident, Dr. Yasmin, yelling at me as he was pushing my mother's stretcher on the way to Radiology for a CT scan. "You better hope your mother doesn't need surgery because we're busy. We won't be able to operate for at least another twelve hours. We wanted to do this CT scan at 6 a.m., and your brother refused. Now it is 4 p.m. and you want it? We don't have time for this."

"My brother refused the CT because my mother was writhing in pain," I shot back. "We have been asking for pain control for three days, and no one has changed her pain meds. Her stomach is more distended and rock hard. Hasn't anyone checked on her in the last twelve hours?"

Eventually, Dr. Silvers met my mother and me in the holding area as we were waiting to have the CT scan.

"Honey, where does it hurt? Honey, you have to quit moaning and tell me where it hurts," Dr. Silvers said, pressing on Mom's distended belly.

Agitated, I answered, "Her name is Ruth. She has a hard time talking because she is in so much pain and short of breath. Can't she get some pain meds?"

Dr. Silvers, surrounded by three residents, yelled in response, "You know, we need to get something straight. Either I manage your mother's care or you do. I don't have time for this. We wanted this scan at 6 a.m."

"Well, if you had done your job, I wouldn't have to. My mom has been writhing in pain for three days. You were told that repeatedly and did nothing," I rebutted.

I wanted to fire Dr. Silvers at that moment. Her behavior was unacceptable. However, I knew that changing surgeons this late in the game could complicate and confuse things for Mom even more. Dr. Silvers was reportedly a good surgeon, although fellow doctors and nurses labeled her as difficult and avoided dealing with her. I knew our family could survive Dr. Silvers for the few weeks Mom would be under her care. We could manage, in order to get a good surgical outcome. But I wasn't going to back down to bully behavior.

Back in Mom's room, we were still waiting for the CT results two hours after the scan. Knowing these results were available immediately in situations like my mother's, I asked the charge nurse, Lynn, to page Dr. Silvers. Lynn's eyes widened and she said, "You're kidding, right? Please don't ask me to do that, Ruth."

"I'm sorry, Lynn, but you and I both know I should have the results by now. Silvers is punishing me by not sharing the results. I need to know if my mom needs surgery. If she does, and they can't perform the surgery here at the community hospital, I need to have her transferred to the trauma center. I'll page Silvers myself if you are afraid to page her."

"No, I'll call her. My shift is almost over anyway. If she screams at me, at least I'm heading out the door. No one ever wants to call her."

Mom did indeed need surgery. Dr. Silvers operated the following morning. Dr. Silvers spoke to my family after the operation and proceeded to tell us what a good job she—Dr. Silvers—had done. She smiled as she said to my family, "You all don't have to like me as long as I'm a good surgeon."

During the next week, we would see Dr. Silvers as she checked on my mom daily. "Don't you *people* ever go home?" she asked one day, shaking her head.

Because of Dr. Silvers' abrasive manner, those caring for Mom, even other physicians, obviously tried to avoid the surgeon. At one point, I realized that a cardiac physician would prefer to risk a cardiac emergency for my mom rather than interrupt Dr. Silvers with a telephone call. According to a staff member, the two doctors just didn't get along.

Personally, I don't care who gets along with Dr. Silvers and who doesn't. I did care about bully behavior and its effect on the care my mother received. I stood my ground in every case, so Mom would get the respect and prompt attention all patients deserve.

Unfortunately, bullying is a reality in health care. In fact, the American Medical Association (AMA) recognized the problem in 2002 by saying, "Personal conduct, whether verbal or physical, that affects or that potentially may affect patient care negatively constitutes disruptive behaviors" (Longo, 2010). The AMA developed a code of conduct for physicians, identifying disruptive behavior as a significant problem in hospitals.

In a survey of 1,565 nurses, by the Institute for Safe Medication Practices, intimidation by physicians was found to have a negative impact on patient care (Unresolved Disrespectful Behavior, 2013). In this survey, 39% of the nurses reported they sometimes encountered physicians' reluctance or refusal to answer questions or return telephone calls or pages; 40% reported physicians' condescending language or voice intonation; and 42% reported physicians' impatience with questions.

Disruptive behaviors—whether exhibited by physicians, nurses, or other health care workers— threaten patient safety because these behaviors break down communication and collaboration. In a study of 4,539 health care workers, 67% felt there was a link between disruptive behaviors and adverse events; 71% felt there was such a link to medication errors; and 27% felt there was a link to patient mortality (Rosenstein & O'Daniel, 2008).

Although health care organizations claim to have zero tolerance for bully behavior, families and patients need to be aware that it exists. For my mother, having a surgeon whom others feared had a ripple effect. My family was aware of her behavior and took steps to mitigate her actions. We persisted in pursuing our rights to communication and prompt attention in the face of any resistance.

We certainly could have fired Dr. Silvers from Mom's case, but we felt it was more important to continue Mom's plan of care and not disrupt it with a change in doctors. As you navigate the health care system, be on the lookout for bully behavior that demeans your loved one or compromises care. Stand up for your rights; insist on communication. When appropriate, ask for a different provider and/or report disruptive behavior to administrators.

ACTION STEPS FOR YOUR FAMILY

1. COMMIT TO VIGILANCE FOR YOUR LOVED ONE
   Come to grips with the fact that you must navigate a broken health care system, one with poor communication and poor coordination of care. Don't let your guard down.

   You can become exhausted quickly as you try to balance hospital visits with work and personal obligations. In addition, it's natural to trust the expertise of your doctor or other health care specialist. Although this is appropriate, even experts sometimes disagree about treatment protocols. And even the most competent and compassionate health care professional operates in a broken system. In many cases in my mother's journey, it wasn't a caregiver but the hospital system that failed.

   Medical errors happen at every hospital and health care facility in the country. Mistakes happen when you least expect them. Persist in asking questions, observing behavior, and insisting on participating in your loved one's plan of care.

2. LEARN TO CONTROL WHAT YOU CAN CONTROL

    Don't waste time in emotional rage against a broken system. Accept the dysfunction as a given, and use your energy to influence things under your control. Arm yourself with vital information, and don't be afraid to speak up—no matter the backlash. Learn the guidelines for preventing hospital errors by visiting the easy-to-navigate websites that follow.

    - Agency for Healthcare Research and Quality:
        - Visit http://www.ahrq.gov; search "never events."
        - Review safe-surgery guidelines at http://www.ahrq.gov; search "making sure your surgery is safe."
    - Joint Commission, national patient-safety goals: Visit http://www.jointcommission.org; search "national patient safety goals."

    For a summary, see Top Ten Ways to Avoid a Medical Error, later in this chapter.

3. INSIST UPON PROMPT AND THOROUGH COMMUNICATION

    Insist on knowing and participating in your loved one's plan of care. Request a copy of the results of all tests and procedures. When necessary, request that your doctor be paged. If the appropriate health care worker refuses to page the doctor, ask to speak to his or her supervisor. You have a right to receive answers. In the case of never events or adverse events, insist that the incident is reported and that you are informed of the resulting plan of care.

4. REFUSE TO ACCEPT BULLY BEHAVIOR

    All patients and families are entitled to information and deserve to be treated with respect. When a request for information or treatment meets with resistance, ask questions until you understand the resistance. If the reason for resistance is invalid in your opinion, persist or ask for a higher authority. If you feel you are being bullied, stand up to it. If necessary, request a new provider and/or report the behavior to administrators.

Top Ten Ways to Avoid a Medical Error

1. Be present for your loved one, or have a loved one with you if you are the patient. This is the most important thing you can do to ensure better care.

2. Demand that all providers wash their hands.

3. Demand that all providers check the patient's ID band before giving any medication or conducting any procedure or interaction with the patient.

4. Demand to be included in the patient's plan of care. This includes being informed of any changes to the plan prior to the change. Remember the definition of patient-centered care: Nothing about me, without me. If a never event or adverse effect occurs, insist that the incident is reported and that you know the resulting plan of care.

5. Know the patient's medications and dosing. Always have a list in your wallet. Question new medications, a change in dosage, or a pill that looks different than usual.

6. Ask for a copy of the results of any procedure and diagnostic test, and keep all copies in your own medical file or binder.

7. Know the name of each provider. Know the role that each provider plays (attending, resident, or intern). Know who the decision makers are in your care (besides you).

Here's a quick rundown of the levels of physician providers:

- A *resident* is in a training program in a medical specialty. The program lasts at least three years.
- An *intern* is in the first year of training after medical school. The first year of training, called *internship*, is also called the *first-year residency,* or *PGY-1* (*postgraduate year 1*). The following years of training are called *second-year residency* (*PGY-2*), *third-year residency* (*PGY-3*), etc.
- A *fellow* is in post residency training (a *fellow-ship*), which is usually training in a specialty. Examples of specialties requiring a fellowship are cardiology, neurosurgery, critical care medicine, etc. All fellows require the supervision of an attending physician.
- An *attending physician* is a doctor who has completed residency training and fellowship (if required for a specialty). An attending physician can practice medicine on his or her own. In most states, when a medical doctor has achieved the attending-physician stage, he or she receives a medical license.

8. Be flexible. Be aware of the hill you'll die on and the ones you won't. Acknowledge that the goal is always quality care. You may have to deal with disruptive

health care providers at times. Decide whether the care each provides is worth the disruptive behavior. Set boundaries. If the result is not quality care, fire the provider from the case.

9. Be informed. Use the Internet to perform your own research. Read the information packet given to you at the hospital. Know your rights as a patient; they must be posted on every floor in the hospital.

10. Speak up! Never be afraid to speak up, ask a question, or challenge something that doesn't look right. Odds are, if something doesn't look right, it isn't right.

CHAPTER 6

MOVE SUCCESSFULLY ACROSS THE CARE CONTINUUM

> *First they ignore you, then they laugh at you,*
> *then they fight you, then you win.*
> ~ Mahatma Gandhi

"YOUR MOM WILL NEED TO LEAVE the ICU and go to an LTAC facility while she weans from the ventilator. The beds there tend to fill up fast, but one will be available at Sunrise Long-Term Care at the end of the week. Our pulmonologists see patients there. If you agree to send your mom to Sunrise, we can get the paperwork started so the bed can be reserved for her," stated Margie, the ICU case manager, while hurriedly leafing through the pile of papers.

I responded, "I understand there are actually three LTAC facilities in the city that take ventilators, right? We'd like to visit all three before deciding on a specific one for my mom. Obviously, I would like to have the same pulmonologist continue to care for my mother, but there are other things to consider as well. My brother, Rick, and I will go check out the facilities," I responded.

"The beds tend to go fast, so it's important that you act quickly," Margie warned. "I can make an appointment for you to visit the facility. Is tomorrow okay?" I agreed to the appointment, understanding that Margie might be pushing the Sunrise facility because the hospital pulmonology team had a contract there.

Rick and I pulled the car into the underground garage of Sunrise, which was littered with windblown garbage. We entered the facility and met with Gerry, the patient liaison, in her sterile, cramped office. Piles of papers were everywhere. We sat around a small round table, barely able to fit the three of us. I had prepared a number of questions for this meeting.

"What's your success rate with ventilator weaning?" I asked.

"I'm really not sure. I'll have to check on that," Gerry answered.

"What is your nurse-to-patient ratio on the ventilator unit?"

"Oh, it is 1:4. We have excellent ratios."

"Is the ratio 1:4 on dayshift only or twenty-four hours a day?"

"Ah, no. The ratio is 1:6 in the evening."

"What is it from 11 p.m. to 7 a.m.?"

"I believe it is 1:8."

"What's your skill mix?" I asked.

"I'm not exactly sure what you mean by that," she replied nervously.

"I want to know how many registered nurses, licensed practical nurses, and nursing assistants you have per shift. I am sure you do not staff your facility with all RNs. I am just wondering how many RNs actually work per shift, compared to LPNs and NAs.

Also, I see you have a recurring advertisement to hire nurses in the Sunday paper. I know you are short-staffed. It's rare to find a hospital that isn't hiring nurses. I know it's even more difficult to hire nurses for an LTAC facility."

"Everyone is looking to hire nurses these days," Gerry defended.

"How many nurses are you short? What's your vacancy rate?"

Rick gave me *the look*. Yes, I sounded like a nurse because I am a nurse! Nurse-to-patient ratios and skill mix have a big influence on the care a patient receives at any facility. I wanted the best for my mom.

As a liaison, Gerry should have known the answers to my questions. This was a for-profit facility, and she didn't have the needed information to make a sale. I needed to know how successful this facility was at doing its job. In my mom's case, the job included weaning a patient from a ventilator. I needed to know if they had the personnel—twenty-four hours a day, seven days a week—to care properly for Mom.

I had an advantage in this interview because I knew the data that described the hospital where I worked. I knew the hospital ran an 80/20 skill mix. This means that at least 80% of direct caregivers on every shift were RNs and 20% were LPNs or NAs.

Registered nurses have more education than LPNs and therefore are able to perform a higher level of nursing care, such as administering certain IV medications. RNs have a higher level of assessment skill than LPNs, which helps permit quick identification of a new problem. NAs are not licensed. The care they are qualified to perform is at a level lower than the care RNs or LPNs perform.

I wanted to know the nurse vacancy rate at Sunrise. The nurse vacancy rate at the hospital where I worked was low, less than 4%. Why is this important? Health care facility administrators determine how many nurses they need based on how many beds they have as well as the type of patients they care for. If a hospital needs 600 nurses to care for all its patients and it has a 4% vacancy rate, they are short 24 nurses out of the 600 they need to operate properly.

Similarly, if a facility that needs 100 nurses to operate has a 30% vacancy rate, it is short 30 nurses out of the 100 nurses needed to operate properly. This was the case at Sunrise, the LTAC facility recommended by the community hospital. Sunrise had a 30% vacancy rate. The facility had only 70% of the nurses needed to care for patients properly.

I learned also that, although the caregiver-patient ratio was supposed to be 1:8 at night, there was actually only one RN or LPN on a floor with 24 to 30 patients. The rest of the caregivers were nursing assistants. Nursing assistants aren't qualified to give medications, assess a patient's condition, or suction lungs. Patients at Sunrise were relying on ventilators to breathe, but the facility had only one licensed nursing staff member in a unit at night. Heaven forbid there was an emergency.

At my request, the respiratory therapist at Sunrise met with us to discuss Sunrise's success with ventilator weaning. He reported that Sunrise had a 70% success rate compared to other hospitals. With further questioning, I learned that this facility benchmarked itself against other facilities, in different states, owned by the same company. I was aghast. Benchmarking against yourself doesn't indicate success on any level, since you all follow the same protocols and processes, which are not necessarily best practices.

Next, I asked Gerry if we could tour the facility. As she walked us through the building, I came upon a glass-enclosed bulletin board full of graphs with quality data. Nursing facilities are required to have their quality data available to residents and patients.

Gerry was quick to point out that I was looking at old data, no longer relevant since they had improved significantly since the reporting. Unfortunately, I didn't see evidence of the improvement. She escorted us to the cafeteria, where she offered to buy us lunch. We left without lunch, since we had seen enough.

Later that day, I saw Dr. Santini, Mom's pulmonologist, at the hospital. He asked how I liked Sunrise. He expected us to have Mom transferred there for ventilator weaning.

"She won't be going to Sunrise," I replied. "Rick and I will be going to check out another LTAC facility tomorrow." We had decided not to visit the third LTAC facility because it had semiprivate rooms. Mom had had enough trouble with infections, even when she was in private rooms. We didn't need the added infection risk of a semiprivate room.

"Why? We can continue to care for her at Sunrise," Dr. Santini said. "We'll take good care of her."

"With all due respect," I returned, "it's not the medical care I am worried about. You and your team do a great job, but you see Mom for only ten minutes a day. I am worried about the other twenty-three hours and fifty

minutes. Sunrise is drastically short of nurses. The facility isn't even using agency nurses to make up the slack.
The facility is running with nursing assistants, mostly. It
is unsafe. How can I send my mother there? Sunrise can't
care for someone on a ventilator. Would you send your
mom there?"

The doctor paused and looked at the floor. "No, Ruth.
I wouldn't. I didn't know Sunrise needed nurses that
badly. I mean, I knew Sunrise was hiring, but I didn't
know the situation was that bad. It sounds unsafe. My
team and I contracted with Sunrise to provide pulmo-
nary services to patients there a few months ago. The
case managers here at the hospital advocate for a lot of
the patients from the hospital to be transferred there
because of continuity of care. I didn't realize Sunrise was
having problems."

The following day, Rick and I headed to another facility, Wholecare Long Term Care. Fearful of what we
might find, we prepared for the worst.

The vibe at Wholecare was totally different from that
at Sunrise. Staff at Wholecare knew we had a *choice* of
facilities. They treated us accordingly.

We met the Wholecare patient liaison, Diane, in the
lobby. She escorted us to her office, where she obviously
would deliver her pitch. The large office looked like an
excerpt from *Better Homes and Gardens.*

I asked Diane the same questions I had asked the liaison at Sunrise. Diane knew the answer to all but one
question, and she immediately picked up the telephone
to find that answer. The nurse-patient ratio at Wholecare
was 1:4 from 7 a.m. to 7 p.m. and 1:6 from 7 p.m. to 7
a.m. The skill mix was 60/40, and the vacancy rate was
12%. Diane was quick to point out that Wholecare was

using agency nurses to staff their facility until they hired more nurses. As a nurse, I knew that this facility, despite being a for-profit business, had a reputation for paying nurses well, so Wholecare was usually able to find agency nurses quickly, to fill open shifts.

Diane took us on a tour of the facility. As we walked down the hall, we passed a bulletin board. Like the bulletin board at Sunrise, this one presented data about the quality of care. I stopped to read the information. Diane began to discuss the data. She highlighted the areas in which Wholecare excelled and acknowledged the areas in which they were deficient. She elaborated on the plan Wholecare had to improve weak areas. We moved on to the next bulletin board, which highlighted wound care. Diane spoke of Wholecare's plastic surgeon, Dr. Blackwell, and the fact the he was well known in the city for his medical management of bedsores.

We asked about Wholecare's success rate with ventilator weaning. In reply, Diane reviewed Wholecare's website with us. We asked about the results of the last inspection, and Diane promised to get the report for us. I had, however, already reviewed all of their data. Reports of inspections are public knowledge and available on Medicare's website, http://www.medicare.gov; search "Nursing Home Compare." This resource allows you to compare nursing facilities in any city in the United States. The site tells you in which areas of care a facility is deficient.

Some of the data on the Medicare site is reported by the facility itself. Other data is the result of an onsite inspection. After reviewing Wholecare's data with me, Diane added, "We certainly aren't perfect, but we know the areas that we need to work on. We have plans in place and are continually improving. I'll be happy to answer any question you have. If I don't know the answer, I will find it."

Next, we toured the High Observation Unit, where my mom would be a patient. All of the patients in this unit were on ventilators. The care mirrored an ICU environment, but the focus here was on ventilator weaning.

I asked Diane, "What was your fall rate last month?"

"Zero. We didn't have any falls last month. It was a good month."

"Then, I need to ask, what is your restraint rate? It's unusual not to have any falls with a patient population like yours."

"It is rare that we restrain someone. Our rate is less than 1%. You know, we have to report that to the state, so we pay close attention to the fall rate and our restraint rate."

"Do you have open visiting hours? I don't see any visitors here right now. That's odd for 12 noon."

"We do have open visiting. Most of our families work during the day. We are full of visitors at night."

Wholecare wasn't perfect, but no place is. Poor staffing is the number one reason for suboptimal care in any LTAC facility. At least Wholecare used agency nurses to supplement its own staff.

We had to make a decision, and this was the better of the two choices. We chose to place Mom in Wholecare and would probably choose the facility again if we had to do it over. Mom was there for only one month before she was transferred back to the hospital, after losing consciousness while getting back to bed. During the month Mom was in Wholecare, she made a lot of headway in weaning from the ventilator. She was doing so well at Wholecare, we assumed that she would be discharged to home from there.

Dr. Donald Berwick, former administrator of the Centers for Medicare and Medicaid Services, refers to *discharge* as a dirty word. He thinks the word *discharge* isn't compatible with patient centeredness (Berwick, 2004).

The mere notion of a discharge implies cutting off all ties. The word also implies an end to the illness or situation that brought the patient to the hospital. In reality, health care facilities should be planning and held responsible for a transition, not a discharge. Decisions concerning transitional care and follow-up care should be carefully considered. The wrong decisions could easily result in a readmission to the hospital.

Currently, health care is converting to a system that will financially penalize hospitals if a patient returns with the same diagnosis within thirty days. Perhaps this incentive will force hospital administrators to view hospitals as having more of a responsibility in transitioning patients to the community.

Most hospitals deliver acute care only. Ideally, after a stay at an acute care hospital, patients are discharged to home. However, many patients need some level of assistance before regaining their optimal level of functioning. If minimal assistance is needed, most patients ask for home care. Some need a little more assistance than home care can provide and opt for an assisted-living facility instead. Patients with more complex needs can be discharged to an appropriate nursing facility.

Various facilities might be appropriate for a patient, depending on his or her medical condition. The options can be confusing, so it is important to understand the differences between them.

Nursing facilities provide one or more of the following types of services:

- Long-term acute care (LTAC), such as health care and services that are needed for an extended period and not available in the typical nursing home or home care environment
- Skilled nursing and medical care and related services
- Rehabilitation (rehab) services that are needed due to injury, disability, or illness

LTAC facilities are certified as acute care hospitals that focus on patients who, on average, are expected to stay approximately twenty-five days. Many patients in LTAC facilities are transferred there from an ICU. LTAC facilities specialize in treating patients who have complex disease processes and require the advantage of an extended hospital stay for treatment.

Many LTAC patients require ventilator weaning, the type of care my mother received. These patients benefit from the intensive respiratory therapy support they receive in this type of facility. Patients with other conditions, such as a traumatic brain injury (TBI), stroke, or complicated organ transplants are often placed in an LTAC to receive rehab as well as respiratory support.

Skilled nursing facilities (SNFs), or nursing homes, provide various levels of medical and nursing care. A licensed physician supervises each patient's care. Skilled nursing care is available on-site, usually twenty-four hours a day. Other medical professionals, such as occupational and physical therapists, are also available. This allows the delivery of medical procedures and therapies on-site, delivery that would not be possible in other facilities. Many patients go to a nursing home for a short period while recovering from a severe wound, amputation, or prolonged surgical or medical stay in a hospital. For many patients, SNF facilities can serve as a good transition between hospital and home.

Rehabilitation facilities are similar to SNFs except their focus of care is on improving a person's physical function. Rehab facilities include medical and nursing care, plus a team of therapists to assist the patient in regaining optimal function. Staff members of rehab facilities care for patients of all ages and conditions. Any patient who is weak, is deconditioned, and/or requires intense physical therapy is a candidate for rehab. However, to qualify for a rehab facility, the patient must be able to tolerate therapy for at least three hours per day. This is a limitation for many patients, particularly the elderly.

Patients who do not qualify for the nursing facilities described so far still have options for care beyond what their families can provide. Assisted-living facilities are an option for individuals who need assistance with activities of daily living (known as ADLs). Services include administration of medications as well as custodial care. In this context, custodial services include assistance with feeding, bathing, and dressing. Many assisted-living facilities are associated with nursing homes so that frail individuals can easily progress across the care continuum when needed.

Home care delivery services are available for patients who are well enough to live at home if they have assistance. The services a person may need range from

simple housekeeping and help with ADLs to nursing
visits and medication management. In addition, various
types of therapy—such as speech, occupational, or physical therapy—can be performed in the home.

Home health aides provide custodial care in home
settings, and their duties are similar to those of nursing
assistants in a hospital. Independent for-profit home care
agencies, hospital agencies, and hospital departments
employ professionals (nurses and therapists) who deliver
care to patients in their homes.

Home care delivery services provided by Medicare-
certified agencies are tightly regulated. For example, one
requirement maintains that a patient must be home-
bound to be able to receive Medicare-reimbursed home
care services. Private insurance companies and HMOs
also have criteria concerning the number of visits covered for specific conditions and services. Restrictions on
the payment source, the physician's orders, and the patient's needs determine the length and scope of services
covered.

Home care nursing services are provided on a part-
time basis. Patients, family members, friends, and other
caregivers are encouraged and taught to handle as much
of the care as possible. Some patients and families feel
they need home care for more hours than Medicare or
their insurance company will pay. In these cases, the
patient or family members must hire a caregiver from a
nursing agency and pay for the caregiver's services
themselves.

The issue here goes beyond payment boundaries; it
extends to the amount of responsibility the patient and
his or her family or caregivers are willing or able to
assume to reach expected outcomes (Centers for Medi-

care & Medicaid Services, 2013c). All too often, the patient or family, with no clear picture of the total care
needed, is left to decide on the best option for care.

THE JOB OF CARE COORDINATION ACROSS THE CONTINUUM

Regardless of where a patient receives follow-up care
after a stay in an acute-care hospital, the job of coordinating care falls into the lap of the family or patient. After
the patient leaves the hospital, the family or patient has
the job of relaying crucial medical information to the
new provider. In the case of Mom's transfer to the LTAC
facility, hospital staff summarized two months of medical records in two short pages. Yes, the hospital sent
copies of the records to the LTAC facility, but no one
read them. Instead, they asked my family members for
Mom's medical history.

After a one-week stay in the hospital, when Mom was
discharged from the ICU to home, with a tracheostomy
and a stage IV bedsore, the discharge papers said to
follow up with the doctor. Period. The discharge papers
didn't say anything else. This is a frightening example of
the common gap in care between the end of a hospitalization and the beginning of home care.

When the home care nurse came to admit Mom to
home care, she started from square one, by asking questions. The home care agency, owned by the same hospital system that discharged my mom, had received only
half a page of medical information about my mother.
That was it. Our family was expected to know and provide her medical history.

With the advent of electronic medical records
(EMRs), one would think that the EMR from the hospital

would interface with the EMR from the home care agency, especially since they were owned by the same organization. Instead, each facility operated as a separate entity, a silo, thereby fragmenting care.

My family found it challenging to find the nursing coverage we felt Mom needed at home. The home care agency provided a short visit from a nurse once or twice a week, to assess Mom's overall status, but the agency didn't provide continuous care. Except for these short visits, my family was responsible for Mom's care. We decided to hire nurses to help.

Initially, we hired nurses who had cared for my mom at the hospital. While hospitalized she received excellent care from many nurses. Hiring some of those nurses, handpicked by her, allowed her to progress on the care continuum at home, as initiatives begun in the hospital continued. This allowed Mom to remain at home, at one point for fifteen consecutive months, without a hospital readmission. This process worked because my mom and family could choose her nurses, assuming a level of competency based on the care the chosen nurses had provided during Mom's hospital stay.

My mom qualified for a county program through the Area Agency on Aging. The program, called Options, gave her six hours of nonskilled care per week. We expected an aide to come to the home and bathe Mom, grocery shop, do laundry, and perform light housekeeping. I was thrilled because the program meant someone else could handle the task of grocery shopping.

Unfortunately, Mom never received these benefits because the agency with which the county contracted could not find enough employees to care for its patient caseload. Although the agency should have refused to take on more patients because of insufficient staffing, they continued to accept additional patients.

At the time of this writing, the agency is paid an average of $17 for every hour of care one of its employees provides; however, the employee gets paid an average of $10 per hour. The job of a nursing assistant is difficult work. Unfortunately, the same person can work in a fast-food restaurant for more money. Therefore, agencies are always short-staffed. The agency is always hiring nurses and aides, so they accept patients with the hope of hiring employees in the interim.

Under the Options program, Mom received about eight hours of service over the course of six weeks. She was entitled to receive forty-eight hours during this time, but the organization didn't have anyone to send to the home.

I spoke to the director and was told that the agency was short-staffed. I asked her how this could happen, when elders relied on them for bathing and weekly shopping. She said the agency tried to rotate staff and send someone to a home at least every other week for a few hours to bathe a patient and buy some groceries. No patient ever received his or her full allotment of hours every week. I was appalled and outraged by this.

This is a county program, and our seniors depend on it. Fortunately, my mom had someone to shop for her and bathe her if someone didn't come, but this is not the case for everyone. Because the program looked good on paper, no one seemed to care.

While Mom was receiving limited services from the county, her Medicaid application was approved and we expected things to get better. Mom was now approved to receive skilled nursing care for sixteen hours per day, seven days a week. We were put in touch with a nursing agency that was quick to tell us they had the nurses to staff an acute case like Mom's. We quickly learned, however, that the nursing agency was also short-staffed. Although at that time the state of Pennsylvania paid the agency $48 for every hour of nursing care it provided, the agency only paid the nurses $21 an hour. The agency had a hard time hiring any nurses, let alone quality nurses, for $21 per hour when hospitals paid a new nurse, without any experience, $22.50 per hour.

In fact, the three part-time nurses I hired from the hospital had to become agency employees if I wanted Medicaid to pay their wages. I battled with the agency to pay these nurses more. After all, they were oriented to Mom's case. The agency didn't have to do anything but provide liability insurance. In this instance, the agency made $27 for every hour Mom received care, and agency personnel had done nothing to recruit the nurses. The agency finally agreed to increase the nurses' pay, but only after I threatened to fire the agency. As it turned out, my mother received care from only one nurse recruited by the agency; I had recruited all the others. To get Medicaid to pay for the services Mom needed, I had to accept this system.

Despite it all, the nursing agency never was able to staff my mom's case and provide care for sixteen hours per day. I wrote letters to the governor and the Department of Human Services, asking for a change in policy. I advocated for allowing families to hire their own nurses as independent contractors if they chose. I argued that, if I could increase the pay to $30 per hour, I would have a better chance of finding experienced nurses. Not only that, experienced nurses could give my mom better care, perhaps avoiding a readmission.

According to my calculations, I could have saved the state of Pennsylvania $100,000 per year, just on my mother's case alone. Marian, Mom's case manager, understood what I was trying to do and agreed that something had to change. In June 2012, Marian asked Rick and me to speak in front of officials of Pennsylvania's Area Agency on Aging. These officials, preparing the following year's budget, were seeking feedback about their services and trying to plan for the onslaught of baby boomers requiring care. Their goal was eventually to allow for care customization; however, they had a ways to go. Although none of the future changes in state funding will affect my mom, I hope the officials do make changes based on our recommendations.

Despite the many downsides of nursing agencies, the services they provide are needed. Certainly, many families would opt to obtain nurses through an agency instead of hiring nurses themselves. Agencies complete background checks, verify credentials, and provide malpractice insurance.

However, I have witnessed nurses placing their own parents into nursing homes because they could not afford to hire someone to care for them or afford to quit their jobs to provide the care themselves. Even though they were nurses, the state would not consider paying them to provide licensed nursing care to their loved ones. We need to think out of the box and individualize care based on the situation. Customization of care must be brought to the forefront as the baby boomers create an "aging tsunami."

* * * * * * *

Throughout my mother's long illness, one link in the continuum of care worked as it should. My mom's PCP, Dr. Farrell, was a constant support and resource. Dr. Farrell knew it was an ordeal to get Mom to his office, so he didn't make her come. Instead, he allowed me to call the office to talk with him when there was an issue.

Dr. Farrell's accessibility made the coordination of care much easier. He acknowledged that my family knew Mom better than anyone did. In fact, he embraced our knowledge and never professed to know more about my mom's illness and journey than we did. We were living this journey, and Dr. Farrell respected that. He knew also that Dr. Belista, Mom's nephrologist, saw Mom every month and ordered lab work. He knew that she was being well cared for and that his job at this point was to help the family coordinate her care.

At one point, it had been nearly one year since Dr. Farrell had examined my mom. His office called, asking if I could bring her in. Mom said, "Absolutely not! If he wants to see me, he can come here or we can FaceTime. I'm not going into his office with all of those sick people."

Dr. Farrell didn't know how to use FaceTime technology. Instead, he packed his weathered black bag and came to my home to assess Mom. Choose your PCP based on your needs, not theirs. Some PCPs are known in the community for embracing the elderly and their desire to age in their own homes. Make sure your PCP knows what your loved one wants and supports those decisions. Having the right PCP can make the difference between staying at home and going to a nursing facility.

* * * * * * *

Although this chapter is about navigating the continuum of care, I would be remiss if I didn't discuss the im-
portance of choosing the appropriate hospital. By now,
you should be painfully aware that medical errors happen at all hospitals. Sometimes, however, you or your
loved one will have a better chance of a good outcome at
one hospital than another, based on the expertise at the
hospital.

Patients choose hospitals for various reasons. Some
want free parking. Others want private rooms. Sometimes the choice of hospital doesn't matter, but oftentimes it does. My mother began her journey at a community hospital. Both of my parents always had an affin-
ity for this hospital because it was close to their home,
parking is cheap and convenient, and patients have private rooms. Although it is a teaching hospital, its primary focus is family practice medicine. The hospital does
not have the same resources that the large trauma center
nearby does.

The community hospital might have to delay an operation because all the operating rooms are in use. This
doesn't happen at a trauma center. Trauma accreditation
is based on the ability to handle multiple acute situations
at one time, and quickly. If you feel that your loved one
is getting sicker and is perhaps too sick for your community hospital, consider a transfer to a larger hospital.
Initiate a conversation with the PCP.

Most doctors won't be offended by this request because they do want the best care possible for the patient.
In many cases, a doctor will suggest a transfer, if he or
she thinks the patient will be better served elsewhere.

This doesn't mean that the doctor isn't knowledgeable. In fact, it can mean the total opposite. Doctors know their limits based on their experience and available resources.

Regardless of the patient's medical condition (be it cancer, an orthopedic problem, complicated surgery, etc.), choose a hospital based on the resources the patient needs.

ACTION STEPS FOR YOUR FAMILY

CHOOSE THE NEXT STEP ON THE CONTINUUM CAREFULLY

1. **DON'T LET A HOSPITAL RUSH YOU**
   Hospitals receive a flat fee for any given diagnosis. After a patient has exceeded the number of hospital days covered by the flat fee, the hospital begins to lose money. The case manager or social worker employed by the hospital will inform you that you have 48 to 72 hours to find a different facility and leave. This is a hospital rule based on finances.

   You have a right to receive the appropriate time needed to find a place that can provide optimal care. Ask your case manager for a list of facilities covered by your insurance company. Explore your options. By law, you are entitled to choose the health care facility that you want to deliver care. You will need to sign a paper indicating that you had freedom of choice before leaving the hospital.

2. **CHOOSE A PROVIDER BASED ON THE PROVIDER'S EXPERTISE**
   Choose your facility or health care professional as if it is a matter of life and death, because many times it will be. Is the hospital considered a "Center of Excellence" by an external standard? Is it a Level I trauma

center? How many knee surgeries does it perform each year? How many gallbladder surgeries does the surgeon perform each year, if gallbladder surgery is the issue?

There is a strong correlation between repetition and competency. It's safe to say that a surgeon who performs the same surgery or procedure 500 times per year will yield better outcomes than one who does the same procedure 10 times per year. In addition to achieving proficiency in the procedure, the provider tends to be better equipped to deal with any complications.

Many cancer patients opt to be treated at a community hospital because it is convenient. Many research studies clearly show that patient outcomes are better at cancer centers than at community hospitals. Health care is very specialized, and it is unrealistic to expect the same level of care from a PCP at a community hospital than from a specialist at a facility that focuses on a specific disease.

3. CHECK FOR RELATIONSHIPS
   If a hospital is recommending a specific facility, find out if the hospital has any relationship to it, financial or otherwise. By law, a hospital must disclose any financial interest it has with another facility. This information can usually be found on the website of the facility. Also, don't be timid about asking direct questions.

4. USE A CHECKLIST
   At the end of this chapter is a checklist of questions to ask and observations to make when visiting a facility. When you visit, you have an obligation to

yourself and your loved ones to assess the safety and the quality of care that facility can deliver. Do not apologize for asking questions or using a checklist during this assessment.

The best facilities will be prepared to answer your questions and provide the information you need to make an informed choice. If a facility is reluctant or unable to answer your questions, treat that as a red flag. Although no place is perfect, withholding information or failing to disclose all of the information tells you an institution can't be trusted. You have a right to be an informed partner in your loved one's or your own care.

REMAIN PROACTIVE IN YOUR RELATIONSHIP WITH LONG-TERM CARE FACILITIES

1. VISIT YOUR LOVED ONE PURPOSEFULLY
    Visit your loved one often, and at various times. Make frequent surprise visits. Be sure to visit at mealtimes and on weekends. Typically, administrators or marketers aren't in the facility on weekends, so you can truly observe the type of care your loved one is receiving. Observe closely whether patients are being fed or assisted by nursing personnel. If the dietary needs of patients are not being met, you have an indicator that other needs aren't being met as well.

2. ELECT ONE FAMILY MEMBER TO BE THE CONTACT POINT
    Communication is more reliable if one person is the contact point throughout the care continuum, be it at the hospital or nursing home. This reduces confu-

sion and prevents misunderstandings and delays in receiving important information.

3. BE AWARE OF ACTUAL MEDICAL CARE

   Your loved one will see a doctor less often in a long-term care facility than in a hospital. In an LTAC facility, most patients usually see a doctor once a day or a few times per week. In a nursing home, the patient will see a doctor once a month. Most nurse-physician interaction concerning patient care takes place over the telephone. If you believe your loved one needs assessment by a doctor, insist on it.

4. TAKE PRECAUTIONS WITH VALUABLES

   Theft and loss are a big concern in nursing homes. Make sure all the patient's belongings have his or her name on them and all items are listed in the inventory that accompanies the patient's chart.

5. KEEP HOSPICE IN MIND

   If you would like your loved one to receive care from a hospice while in a nursing home, hospice care may be an option. However, many nursing homes do not share this information because the nursing home will lose a portion of reimbursement to the hospice provider.

6. SPEAK UP!

   If you are not happy with the care that your loved one is receiving, speak up! Give the facility a chance to rectify the issues. If the issues are not taken care of, remember that you can have your loved one transferred to another facility. Also remember that the care at a nursing home or LTAC facility will not be the same care as at a hospital. Each type of facility provides a different level of care.

7. CONTACT YOUR STATE'S LONG-TERM CARE OMBUDSMAN

Every state has a long-term care ombudsman who works to resolve problems of individual residents and bring about changes at the local, state, and national levels to improve residents' care and quality of life. This person is available to answer questions and to advocate for you regarding long-term care issues. All services are free. Information can be found on the website of the Area Agency on Aging in your particular state.

Ombudsmen serve a vital role in the care of patients in long-term care facilities.

The Administration on Aging (2013) reports program data for fiscal year 2011 (the latest data available at this writing). The report indicates that long-term care ombudsman services to residents were provided by 1,186 full-time–equivalent staff and 9,065 volunteers trained and certified to investigate and resolve complaints.

These paid ombudsmen and volunteers:

- Worked to resolve 204,044 complaints, opening 134,775 new cases (a case contains one or more complaints originating from the same source)
- Resolved or partially resolved 73% of all complaints to the satisfaction of the resident or complainant
- Provided 289,668 consultations to individuals
- Visited at least quarterly 70% of all nursing homes and 33% of all board-and-care, assisted-living, and similar homes
- Conducted 5,144 in-facility training sessions on such topics as residents' rights

- Provided 114,033 consultations to long-term
  care facility managers and staff and participated in 20,958 resident council and 3,321 family
  council meetings

In 2012 the most frequent complaints against nursing
facilities involved

- Improper eviction or inadequate discharge
  planning
- Lack of respect for residents, poor staff atti-
  tudes
- Medications (administration and organization)
- Resident conflict, including roommate-to-
  roommate conflict

The five most frequent complaints against board-and-
care homes and similar facilities involved

- Quality, quantity, variation, and choice of food
- Medications (administration and organization)
- Inadequate notice or no planning regarding
  discharge or eviction
- Equipment or building hazards
- Lack of respect for residents, poor staff atti-
  tudes

CHECKLIST FOR ASSESSING LONG-TERM CARE FACILITIES

QUESTION	ADEQUATE?		COMMENT
	Y	N	
Is the staffing ratio for the level of care your loved one needs adequate?			
How many of the above caregivers are RN's?			
How many of the above caregivers are LPN's?			
What is the current vacancy rate for nursing?			
Do they supplement nursing staff with agency nurses?			
For agency nurses, how long is their orientation to the facility?			
How many patients fell in the past month?			
What was the restraint rate last month (%)?			
How many of the patients developed a bedsore last month?			
What is their standard protocol for preventing bedsores?			
How often do they turn all of their patients or change their position?			

QUESTION	ADEQUATE?		COMMENT
	Y	N	
Take note of the noise level of the facility. Is it loud? Are patients screaming?			
How does it smell? Can you smell urine?			
How often do you have patient care meetings?			
Can family attend all patient care meetings?			
What happens in the event of a medical emergency?			
Do you encourage patients to bring personal belongings from home?			
Have you had a problem with theft of personal belongings in the past?			
When was your last inspection? (Note that the internet has this info also.)			
How much input does the patient have concerning their daily routine?			
Is this a Patient-Centered Care facility?			

CHAPTER 7

NAVIGATE INSURANCE, MEDICARE, MEDICAID, AND VA BENEFITS

> *When walking alone in a jungle of true dark-*
> *ness, there are three things that can show you*
> *the way: instinct to survive, the knowledge of*
> *navigation, creative imagination. Without them,*
> *you are lost.*
>
> ~ Toba Beta,
> My Ancestor Was an Ancient Astronaut

WHEN YOU ATTEMPT TO NAVIGATE any government-subsidized program or private insurance company, you quickly realize you are walking in a jungle of true darkness. Regardless of background, most patients and families find the experience overwhelming and confusing. I have seen families give up the fight to gain approval for services because they could not take on one more battle. As with most things in life, perseverance is the key in navigating the complex and foreign world of health care.

When Mom became seriously ill, I realized quickly that I would need a basic understanding of insurance programs to navigate them effectively. I began my quest to understand these complex areas. My hope was to gain just enough knowledge to ensure Mom's private insurance company and Medicare (and eventually Medicaid) would approve and cover her medical treatments. My journey for more knowledge began with an inquiry into the history of these programs.

American Medical insurance began in 1929, when Justin Ford Kimball, an administrator at Baylor University Hospital in Dallas, Texas, realized that many schoolteachers were not paying their medical bills. In response to this problem, he developed the Baylor Plan. Under this plan, teachers paid 50 cents per month in exchange for the guarantee they could receive medical services when needed (Blumberg & Davidson, 2009).

With the onset of the Great Depression, in the 1930s, many hospitals followed the model of the Baylor Plan, and medical insurance became widespread. Prepaid health plans enabled consumers to be insured. The plans benefited hospitals by supplying steady income despite economic turmoil. However, these single-hospital plans generated price competition.

To address this, community hospitals started to work together to create health coverage plans. In 1939, the American Hospital Association (AHA) first used the name *Blue Cross* to designate health care plans that met AHA standards. In 1960, these plans merged under AHA to form Blue Cross.

Prepaid plans covering the services of physicians and surgeons also began to emerge. These were physician-sponsored plans, and in 1946, they eventually combined to form Blue Shield. Blue Cross and Blue Shield merged into one company in 1971.

The government didn't become involved in health care until the mid-1950s. In 1954, Social Security coverage included disability benefits for the first time. In 1965, the Medicare and Medicaid programs were introduced.

In the 1970s and 1980s, more expensive medical technology and flaws in the health care system led to higher costs for health insurance companies. Responding to these higher costs, employee benefit plans changed into managed care plans and health maintenance organizations (HMOs) emerged (Blumberg & Davidson, 2009).

In 1993, in an attempt to address problems in the U.S. health care system, President Bill Clinton proposed universal health care. Congress rejected the proposal. New developments in health insurance did take place, however, including passage of the Mental Health Parity Act and the Health Insurance Portability and Accountability Act (HIPAA). Both were passed in 1996. However, with the failure of Clinton's proposal for universal health care, there was no fundamental restructuring of the U.S. health insurance system. In 2010, President Barack Obama signed the Patient Protection and Affordable Care Act, usually known as the Affordable Care Act (ACA). All the changes to health care resulting from the ACA will take years to roll out.

Currently, you can purchase insurance from a private company by paying a specific amount either on a monthly or quarterly basis. The payment is referred to as a premium, and you pay the fee in advance for future coverage benefits.

Typically, when you purchase a health insurance policy, you receive a health insurance identity card to present to a clinic, doctor, or hospital for verification and identification purposes. If you receive care from a direct-claims settlement facility, the provider facility sends the medical expense bill to the insurance company directly, for reimbursement. The provider bills the insurance company directly, and no money or claim form must pass through your hands as the patient.

This process sounds logical and straightforward, but it is complicated by multiple variables. A patient can be denied coverage because of a pre-existing illness or disability. In addition, monthly premiums can cost several hundreds of dollars. Premiums usually increase as a patient's age increases. Historically, women of childbearing age have paid more than men of the same age.

Many employers offer health insurance as a benefit to full-time employees, with the employer paying a portion, if not the majority, of the monthly premium. The cost of the premium is often determined by the size of the employee's company. Larger companies that have a mix of high- and low-risk individuals can negotiate lower overall rates. Many employees who work for smaller companies bear the burden of higher premiums because of high-risk coworkers.

Some employers do not offer any health care insurance benefits, even to full-time employees. These individuals are left to figure out how to pay for health care on their own.

WHAT ARE THE DIFFERENT TYPES OF HEALTH INSURANCE?

Different types of health insurance plans meet different needs. When you compare insurance plan options, understanding how they are structured is important. The Centers for Medicare & Medicaid Services (2013f) provide the information that follows.

HEALTH MAINTENANCE ORGANIZATIONS (HMOS) AND EXCLUSIVE PROVIDER ORGANIZATIONS (EPOS)

HMOs and EPOs may limit coverage to providers inside their networks. A network is a list of doctors, hospitals, and other health care providers that provide medical care to members of a specific health plan. If you use a doctor or facility that isn't in the HMO's network, you may have to pay the full cost of the services provided. HMO members usually have a PCP and must get referrals to see specialists. This is generally not true for EPO members.

PREFERRED-PROVIDER ORGANIZATIONS (PPOS) AND POINT-OF-SERVICE PLANS (POSS)

These insurance plans give you a choice of obtaining care within or outside a provider network. With a PPO or POS plan, you may use out-of-network providers and facilities, but you'll have to pay more than if you use in-network providers or facilities.

HIGH-DEDUCTIBLE HEALTH PLANS (HDHPS)

These plans feature lower premiums and higher deductibles than do traditional insurance plans. As of 2013, HDHPs are plans with a minimum deductible of $1,250 per year for individual coverage and $2,500 for family coverage.

CATASTROPHIC HEALTH INSURANCE PLANS

A catastrophic health insurance plan covers essential health benefits but has a very high deductible. The insurance provides safety-net coverage in case you have an accident or serious illness. Catastrophic plans usually do not provide coverage for prescription drugs, shots, and the like. Premiums for catastrophic plans may be lower than those for traditional health insurance plans, but deductibles are usually much higher. This means you must pay thousands of dollars out-of-pocket before full coverage kicks in.

Affordable Care Act Health Plans

The options and changes in the list that follows are current at the time of publication of this book. The ACA

1. Created the Health Insurance Marketplace, a set of organizations that allow purchase of health insurance under the ACA. One way to access the marketplace is by means of a government website that allows the user to review and choose a health care plan based on options available in his or her state. This represents a new way for individuals, families, and small businesses to obtain health care coverage.

2. Requires insurance companies to cover people who have pre-existing health conditions.

3. Holds insurance companies accountable for rate increases.

4. Makes it illegal for health insurance companies to cancel health insurance arbitrarily, just because the insured gets sick.

5. Protects the patient's right to choose his or her doctors.

6. Allows family insurance plans to cover young adults under age 26.

7. Provides free preventive care.

8. Ends lifetime and yearly dollar limits on coverage of essential health benefits.

9. Guarantees the right to appeal (see Centers for Medicare & Medicaid Services, 2013b).

Every October, *open enrollment* begins for individuals with private insurance and for those covered by Medicare. It is extremely important to investigate options carefully, since they tend to be quite confusing.

Medicare guidelines are especially relevant, even for those who don't have Medicare. Medicare guidelines set the standards for minimum care that all insurance companies, government and private insurers, must meet. Many private insurance companies provide benefits above this level.

How Does Medicare Work?

President Lyndon B. Johnson signed the Medicare and Medicaid programs into law on July 30, 1965. Initially, Medicare and Medicaid were enacted as Title XVIII and Title XIX, respectively, of the Social Security Act. The act extended health coverage to almost all Americans age 65 and older and provided health care services to low-income children deprived of parental support; their caregiver relatives; and the elderly, the blind, and individuals with disabilities. Americans age 65 and older were the demographic group most likely to be living in poverty; before 1965, only about half had insurance coverage. In 1972, Medicare eligibility was extended to individuals under age 65 with long-term disabilities and to individuals with end-stage renal disease.

Medicare was designed as a fee-for-service system. Physicians receive payment based on services they provide to each patient. In other words, the more patients a physician sees, the more money the office makes.

Have you ever wondered why your physician spends only fifteen minutes with you? Have you ever wondered why you have to wait so long in the waiting room to see a physician? The current payment system rewards providers for the patient encounter, not the quality of the encounter. Wouldn't it make sense to reward providers based on the quality of the care they provide? If a provider spends forty-five minutes discussing strategies to reduce the risk of another heart attack with a patient, and the patient is successful in implementing these strategies for change, shouldn't the provider be rewarded? Our current broken medical system is set up to promote volume, not effective, patient-centered care.

Hospitals receive payment based on a patient's specific diagnosis. For example, if a patient is hospitalized for pneumonia, Medicare guidelines authorize a certain number of hospital days for treatment. If a patient exceeds the number of days that Medicare or an insurance company allows for a specific diagnosis, the hospital must absorb the cost. It is not uncommon for a patient to be hospitalized and released, only to be re-hospitalized within thirty days with the same problem. In what other business would this be permitted?

In 2013, Medicare finally began to change its reimbursement structure regarding specific disease processes. Medicare administrators realized they needed to reward providers who work hard at avoiding readmissions. Medicare is now penalizing hospitals that have high thirty-day readmission rates.

Initially, the financial penalty imposed by Medicare will be 1% and will apply to a few diagnoses only, diagnoses such as heart failure, heart attack, and pneumonia. By 2015, the penalty will increase to 3% and apply to seven diagnoses.

In addition, physician payment will be based on value not volume. Payments will be modified so that physicians who provide higher-value care will receive higher payments than those who provide lower-quality care (Health Resources and Services Administration, 2013).

According to the Centers for Medicare & Medicaid Services (2013d), the 2013 Medicare program covers the following:

- People age 65 or older
- People under age 65 with certain disabilities
- People of all ages with end-stage renal disease

PART A: HOSPITAL INSURANCE

Most participants aren't required to pay a premium for Medicare Part A (hospital insurance) because they or a spouse has already paid for this coverage through payroll taxes. Medicare Part A helps cover inpatient care in hospitals and skilled nursing facilities, but not long-term care. It also helps cover hospice care and some home health care.

PART B: MEDICAL INSURANCE

Most participants are required to pay a monthly premium for Medicare Part B (medical insurance). Medicare Part B helps cover doctors' services and outpatient care. It also covers other medical services that Part A doesn't cover, such as some services offered by physical and occupational therapists, and some home health care and medically necessary supplies.

PART C: MEDICARE ADVANTAGE PLAN

A Medicare Advantage Plan (Medicare Part C) is a health plan offered by a private company that contracts with Medicare to provide participants with all Medicare Part A and Part B benefits. A Medicare Advantage Plan can be an HMO, PPO, private fee-for-service plan, special-needs plan, or Medicare Medical Savings Account plan. For participants enrolled in a Medicare Advantage Plan, Medicare services not paid for under Original Medicare are covered through the plan. Most Medicare Advantage Plans also provide prescription drug coverage.

Medicare Advantage Plans work in conjunction with private insurance companies. Each month Medicare pays, to the companies that offer Medicare Advantage Plans, a fixed amount for each participant's care. The companies must follow rules set by Medicare. However, each Medicare Advantage Plan can charge different out-of-pocket costs and have different rules about specific services. For example, a plan might require participants to go, for nonemergency care, to doctors, facilities, or suppliers that belong to the plan. The rules can change each year.

If the plan decides to stop participating in Medicare, participants have to join another Medicare Advantage Plan or return to Original Medicare.

PART D: PRESCRIPTION DRUG COVERAGE

Everyone with Medicare can get prescription drug coverage, which lowers out-of-pocket prescription costs and may help protect the insured against higher drug costs in the future. Most participants must pay a monthly premium for prescription coverage. Medicare Prescription Drug Coverage is provided by private companies. Beneficiaries choose the drug plan.

LONG-TERM CARE

Medicare pays for long-term care only if the participant requires skilled medical services or rehabilitative care. It does not pay for non-skilled assistance with activities of daily living (known as ADLs), which make up the majority of long-term care services. Medicare will pay for a home care visit by a nurse when medically necessary but will not provide around-the-clock care.

OUT-OF-POCKET EXPENSES

If you have Original Medicare, you may consider buying a Medicare supplemental policy known as Medigap. A Medigap policy is health insurance sold by a private insurance company to help pay some of the health care costs that Original Medicare doesn't cover. There are twelve standard Medigap policies (Medigap Plans A through L). Insurers selling Medigap must follow state and federal laws designed to protect you.

If you are enrolled in a Medicare Advantage Plan, you don't need to buy (and can't be sold) a Medigap policy (which is different from a Medicare Advantage Plan). A Medigap policy supplements Original Medicare benefits only.

Many Medicare recipients, regardless of type of policy or supplemental policy, find that they need long-term assistance. Medicare does not pay the largest part of long-term care services or personal care—such as help with bathing or for supervision, often called custodial care. Medicare will help pay for a short stay in a skilled nursing facility, for hospice care, or for home health care if you meet the following conditions:

- You have had a recent hospital stay of at least three days.
- You are admitted to a Medicare-certified nursing facility within thirty days of your hospital stay.
- You need skilled care, such as skilled nursing services, physical therapy, or other types of therapy.

If you meet all these conditions, Medicare will pay for some of your costs for up to 100 days. For the first twenty days, Medicare pays 100% of your costs. For days 21 through 100, you pay your own expenses, up to $140 per day (as of 2013), and Medicare pays any balance. You pay 100% of costs for each day you stay in a skilled nursing facility after day 100.

In addition to skilled-nursing facility services, Medicare pays for the following services, for a limited time, when your doctor says they are medically necessary:

- Part-time or intermittent skilled nursing care.
- Physical therapy, occupational therapy, and speech-language pathology, ordered by your doctor, to be provided by a Medicare-certified home health agency for a limited number of days.
- Medical social services to help cope with the social, psychological, cultural, and medical issues that result from an illness. These may include help accessing services and follow-up care; services that explain how to use health care and other resources; and services that help explain a disease.

- Medical supplies and DME, such as wheel-
  chairs, hospital beds, oxygen, and walkers. For
  DME, you pay 20% of the Medicare-approved
  amount.

As you can see, the cost of health care for an ill Medicare patient can quickly become unmanageable, deplet-
ing already-limited funds. This leads many to seek help
through Medicaid, the government safety-net program.

HOW DOES MEDICAID WORK?

The Medicaid program was enacted to provide health
care services to low-income children deprived of parental
support; their caregiver relatives; and the elderly, the
blind, and individuals with disabilities. Historically, those
who received welfare cash assistance received their
health insurance through the Medicaid program. The
welfare link to Medicaid was eventually severed and
enrollment (or termination) of Medicaid was no longer
automatic with the receipt (or loss) of welfare cash assistance (Centers for Medicare & Medicaid Services, 2013a).
Each state now operates a Medicaid program that provides health coverage for lower-income families and
children, the elderly, and people with disabilities.

Although eligibility rules for Medicaid are different
in each state, most states offer coverage for adults who
have children and an income below a specific level. Beginning in 2014, most adults under age 65 with individual incomes up to about $15,000 per year will qualify for
Medicaid in every state. People with disabilities are eligible in every state. In some states, people with disabilities
qualify automatically if they get Supplemental Security
Income (SSI) benefits. In other states, individuals may

qualify depending on income and resources (financial assets).

Sometimes, in cases of catastrophic illness or accident, the only way to get the treatment needed for a loved one is to apply for Medicaid. Many working and insured individuals struck with a catastrophic illness find themselves unable to work and with mounting debt. Their only recourse is Medicaid. Unfortunately, Medicaid approval can take months, and the delay in approval can be frustrating.

Qualifying for Medicaid

Many individuals assume that their income is too high to qualify for Medicaid. However, after a person subtracts large medical expenses, he or she may fall into a lower income bracket. Many patients and families struggle to pay bills that Medicaid would cover. Each state has different rules about eligibility and applying for Medicaid. Call your state Medicaid program to see if you qualify.

Even if your income exceeds Medicaid income levels in your state, you may be eligible under Medicaid *spend-down rules.* Under the spend-down process, some states allow you to become eligible for Medicaid as *medically needy,* even if you have too much income to qualify. This process allows you to spend down, or subtract, your medical expenses from your income to become eligible for Medicaid. To be eligible as medically needy, your measurable resources must also be under the resource amount allowed in your state. To learn more about the guidelines in your individual state, see Centers for Medicare & Medicaid Services (2013d).

HOW TO PAY FOR HOSPICE CARE

Medicare covers hospice care if you have a terminal illness and are not expected to live for more than six months. If you qualify for hospice services, Medicare covers drugs to control symptoms of the illness and pain relief; medical and support services from a Medicare-approved hospice provider; and other services that Medicare does not otherwise cover, such as grief counseling. You may receive hospice care in your home, in a nursing home (if that is where you live), or in a hospice care facility. Medicare also pays for some short-term hospital stays and inpatient care for caregiver respite.

VETERANS BENEFITS—YOU DON'T HAVE TO BE A VET!

Even individuals who have never served in the military may be eligible for veterans' benefits. For example, a social worker informed me that my mom might be eligible for the Aid and Attendance benefit from the Veterans Administration (VA). This benefit helps to pay for an attendant (nurse or aide) for a person who is unable to care for him- or herself. My father served in World War II, and this benefit extends to spouses as well as veterans. I used the VA website to research this benefit. Mom appeared to be eligible for about $1,100 per month as the spouse of a veteran.

The application process is complicated, and according to the VA website, the average wait for an eligibility decision is approximately six months. If benefits are awarded, however, they are paid retroactively to the time of application.

At many local Veterans of Foreign War (VFW) organizations, at no cost, vets assist other vets and their families with the Aid and Attendance application. Our family made the mistake of hiring a VA-accredited representative who charged $1,000 to expedite Mom's VA benefits. This man was unable to keep his promises, and Mom died before receiving any benefits. If you or your loved one is a veteran or spouse of a veteran of any war, explore this VA benefit. Just be sure to avoid paying for application assistance that you can get free.

LESSONS WE LEARNED ALONG THE WAY

Fortunately, my mother had chosen a Medicare Advantage HMO plan years before falling ill. Although no insurance is perfect, this plan provided her with enhanced medical coverage. As the following accounts illustrate, insurance coverage often plays a significant role in the care you receive.

We feared we would never obtain insurance approval for home dialysis for my mother, but we eventually found a physician and dialysis center willing to accept my mother as a patient. Finally, it appeared that home dialysis would become a reality.

Dr. Belista declared, "I think we can arrange for you to dialyze your mother at home. We've personally never had anyone who has a tracheostomy be on home hemodialysis, and no one I know has ever done it. Still, I am willing to try it. It should definitely improve her quality of life. Home hemodialysis is usually done six days a week. Some patients do it five days a week. Your mom is so small, at 100 pounds and 5 feet tall, that maybe she could do it every other day. However, Medicare requires that patients on home hemodialysis dialyze at least five times a week. The research shows that dialyzing five times weekly produces the best outcome."

"Okay," I answered, "We'll do whatever we have to do to be approved by our insurance company for home hemodialysis. If I have to dialyze six days a week, so be it. So, do you think everything will be approved?"

A reasonable person would think Mom's Medicare Advantage HMO Plan, provided by a private insurance company, would easily approve the home hemodialysis. Research indicates that being dialyzed at home drastically improves a patient's quality of life, since the frequent dialysis treatments more closely mirror normal kidney function. Mom wouldn't have much of the discomfort that resulted from three-times-weekly outpatient dialysis—discomfort that resulted from the huge flux in fluid status and the other changes indicated by shifting lab values. In addition, with home dialysis the potential for infection would decrease, since Mom wouldn't have to go to the hospital for dialysis. Despite all these benefits, two factors complicated things: Mom was 82 years old and had a tracheostomy.

Dr. Belista must have presented a good case. Despite our worries about Medicare approval, Mom was approved for home hemodialysis. Home hemodialysis did exactly what we hoped it would; it drastically improved Mom's quality of life. Her nutritional status improved as well, because her appetite increased. Because of the increased frequency of dialysis, Mom's diet could be more liberal. She could now eat a homegrown tomato with her scrambled eggs, even though tomatoes are high in potassium, because we would be dialyzing that afternoon. Mom's weight went from 100 pounds to 130 pounds in a few months, shocking all of her physicians. Her albumin, an indicator of protein in the human body and necessary for shrinking Mom's bedsore, was normal for the first time in eighteen months. Her bedsore became smaller.

Medicare guidelines required Mom to be dialyzed at least five days a week. Monthly labs checked on how well dialysis was clearing the toxins from her blood. Mom's labs were very good on a five-day-a-week dialysis schedule. Since Mom's labs were so good and she was so small, I asked Dr. Belista if we could try dialysis four days a week.

Dr. Belista cautioned that Medicare had approved the home dialysis based on a five-day-a-week schedule. The doctor wasn't sure how Medicare would respond if we dialyzed four days a week. Despite Dr. Belista's uncertainty, she agreed that we could try a four-day-a-week dialysis schedule and base all decisions on Mom's monthly labs. We followed the labs closely and found that Mom had adequate toxin clearance from the dialysis when it was done four days a week. Because of her size, this schedule yielded an optimal outcome: clearance was good, she reported no adverse signs or symptoms, and she reported a 10/10 quality-of-life score. Despite the revised schedule, we still received supplies based on a five-day-a-week schedule up until she died. Medicare had been informed that we were dialyzing four days a week instead of five, but the supplies continued to be delivered based on the original schedule.

Sometimes, the supposedly easy things can be the most difficult to get approved by an insurance company. At an earlier point in Mom's illness, the insurance company owned by the health system in which Mom was hospitalized was the provider of her Medicare Advantage HMO Plan. When Mom initially needed to be transferred to an LTAC facility for ventilator weaning, after her first ICU stay, she was immediately approved by the HMO.

On another occasion, however, when Mom needed to be transferred back to the LTAC facility from the trauma center (after being admitted there for a brief time following a loss of consciousness)—well, that was a different story. In that instance, the same insurance company refused to approve the transfer. Although Mom again needed to be weaned from the ventilator—and the LTAC facility did this better than the trauma center did—the insurance company denied approval. According to the insurance company, someone of my mother's age and with her multiple disease conditions was not likely to wean; therefore, she was not approved for LTAC. As I mentioned in an earlier chapter, the hospital's solution was for Mom to be transferred to a nursing home, despite the fact that nursing homes are not in the business of weaning patients from a ventilator.

We decided to appeal the decision. We filed an *expedited appeal* with the insurance company. An expedited appeal may be filed if the patient believes his or her life, health, or ability to regain maximum function is in immediate jeopardy. Once an expedited appeal is filed, an insurance company (or Medicare, if that is the case) has seventy-two hours to respond. In our case, the insurance company chose not to render a decision for nearly thirty days. We didn't push for a quick decision, because Mom was still in the ICU.

As we prepared to file the next level of appeal with the Centers for Medicare & Medicaid Services (known as CMS), one of the pulmonologists, Dr. Keister, approached me.

"Ruth, why are you filing a CMS appeal?"

"Mom was denied the LTAC facility, and I don't want her to go to a nursing home. I know everyone says she can't be weaned from the vent, but no one really knows for sure since no one has aggressively tried."

"Well, I want you to stop and think about something. The hospital is not kicking her out. The appeal was denied, and we talked about a nursing home being her best option, but no one is kicking her out of this hospital. Not yet, anyway. You may have lost the battle but not the war. I wouldn't do anything. I would just let her stay here." I thought about it. Why file a CMS appeal unless I had to?

The hospital's stance made sense when viewed in the context of an important fact: The hospital system owned both the trauma center and the insurance company. The system did not own the LTAC facility. This decision, like so many others, had come down to dollars and cents. Why should the health system's hospital pay another facility for services the health system could provide?

At the point the stalemate began to cost the hospital money because Mom's extended stay was outside insurance payment parameters, the ICU began to wean my mother aggressively from the ventilator. Within a month, Mom went from being on the ventilator twenty-four hours a day to eight hours a day. She was finally going to be discharged to home.

Guidelines on Supplies

Our family also had to battle to obtain the supplies Mom needed after she was discharged to home. Hopefully, our story will help you in your quest to obtain the supplies that you need to care for your loved one.

In a prior chapter, I mentioned that Dr. Daniels wrote a prescription for suction catheters. This allowed us to use new rather than repeatedly washed catheters to suction secretions through Mom's tracheostomy. I am certain our vigilant infection-control practices decreased Mom's hospital readmission rate.

In addition to frequent suctioning, my mother required daily dressing changes on her bedsore and on skin tears on her arms. At one point, although I had meant to place my order for dressing supplies a week earlier, I did not place the order until the first day of the month after the usual ordering date.

Unbeknownst to me, the vendor, who had been allowing us to order the supplies whenever we needed them, had changed the rules for ordering. I was instructed that my mom's insurance company (which was providing her Medicare Advantage HMO Plan) was now allotting supplies based on the current Medicare guidelines.

The insurer had sent no letter to patients; it gave no advance warning. Instead, the company changed the rules midstream. This meant we were in a crisis. Mom required three types of dressing supplies just to change her bedsore dressing. The secretary who answered the telephone actually gave advice on how to handle the new rules. The conversation went like this:

"I need to order a thirty-day supply of 2×2s, Nu Gauze, and Mepilex for her bedsore. I also need Mepitel for two skin tears on her arms."

"I can't send you those supplies. You are only allowed to have one dressing supply for each wound. That is the Medicare guideline."

"That can't be right. My mother acquired a stage IV bedsore at the hospital, and now the insurance company, owned by the same hospital system, is telling me I can't get the supplies to perform the dressing change per her doctor's orders?"

"I'm sorry, but other patients who order from us have been doing the dressing change every other day so they don't run out of supplies. You might want to consider that."

"If I'm hearing you correctly, you're telling me to not follow the doctor's orders and change the frequency of the dressing change because you won't send me the supplies I need? Is that what you're telling me?"

"Well, I'm just saying that you might want to consider this. Other patients are doing this to make the supplies last the full month."

"Are you a nurse? "

"No."

"Do you know it is against the law to practice medicine without a license? Can I speak to your wound nurse, please?"

I was furious. I had played by the rules. I had ordered only what I needed every month. I was always careful not to waste supplies. Now I was paying a high price for following the rules.

The wound care nurse informed me that I would have to get a physician's order to obtain more dressing supplies. I informed her that she already had the order and could clearly see that I needed more than one dressing supply for Mom's bedsore. That didn't matter.

The only way for me to get the supplies I needed was to obtain another physician's order that explained why I needed more than one type of dressing for the bedsore. I contacted the physician and faxed the vendor the order. I received the supplies I needed. The game changed that day, and I had learned the hard way. From that day forward, I would never come remotely close to running out of supplies again.

Mom continued with the Medicare Advantage HMO plan from the private insurer, but eventually she applied for Medicaid, to assist with her health care costs. Like many patients and families, we were unable to continue to pay multiple co-pays for visits to doctors, medications, and medical equipment, as well as for the additional nursing care that the Medicare HMO did not cover. We delayed applying for Medicaid because Mom owned part of her home. We didn't want Medicaid acceptance to affect ownership of her house. Eventually, Medicaid became the logical solution for us, however.

Medicaid eligibility involves strict income guidelines as well as guidelines concerning assets. Because these guidelines vary from state to state, be sure to review the Medicaid guidelines for your specific state. You can do this at http://www.medicaid.gov; search "state plan amendments."

As we went through the application process for Medicaid for my mother, our family learned that we needed to request a receipt of delivery for everything we sent to the state. Things had a way of getting lost. Mom was eventually approved for Medicaid and much of the financial burden of her care was lifted.

ACTION STEPS FOR YOUR FAMILY

DEALING WITH INSURANCE, MEDICARE, AND MEDICAID

1. **CHOOSE YOUR INSURANCE POLICY WISELY**

   When choosing an insurance plan, consider the list that follows. Make your decisions after considering how often you expect to utilize health care in the next year, based on your current health. Make sure you understand what the policy does and does not cover. Even if Medicare or Medicaid isn't in your near future, understanding your insurance benefits is crucial to equipping yourself with adequate coverage in case something catastrophic happens.

   - Do your best to balance the cost (monthly premium) of a policy with the protection it offers.

   - Determine what expenses (deductible, co-insurance, co-payments, and out-of-pocket costs) you will have to pay for covered services.

   - Estimate costs for non-covered care (services excluded or limited by the policy).

   - Check that the plan covers the health care services and medications you require.

   - Check whether the plan's health care providers include your current providers, if the providers are convenient to your location, and if the providers are of high quality.

   - Avoid policies that don't have some kind of maximum out-of-pocket limit on covered charges.

   - Be careful not to mistake insurance-like products for comprehensive coverage. Comprehensive medical insurance consists of health insurance that provides coverage for most types of medical expenses.

- Be sure to review the Summary of Benefits and Coverage (SBC) document. A SBC is a summary of the benefits that your plan covers and the cost-sharing ratio (portion the consumer pays) associated with that coverage.

Every insured person should be aware of the terms and conditions of coverage of the health insurance plan he or she purchases. Non-covered items are listed in the exclusion section of the policy document. Some plans:

- Do not cover medical expenses that arise as the result of injuries or accidents due to substance abuse or alcohol addiction.

- Do not cover medical expenses that arise as a result of self-inflicted injuries or suicide attempts.

- Offer full reimbursement only if the patient consults a medical expert, clinic, or hospital tied to its network. Otherwise, the individual may have to bear a certain percentage of the expense.

- Require approval for an elective surgery before a patient can be admitted for the surgery and to enable the patient to receive full reimbursement for related medical expenses.

2. VISIT THE HEALTH INSURANCE MARKETPLACE
    Visit www.healthcare.gov/marketplace/individual/ to
    learn about the insurance options available in your
    state as part of the Affordable Care Act.

    If you are a young person and shopping for yourself,
    don't tempt fate. Many younger individuals do not
    see the need for health insurance, but catastrophic
    events can happen at any age. In addition, practicing
    preventive care (which insurance plans cover) in the
    early years reaps benefits later in life. Maintaining
    your health in your early years can translate into
    lower premiums and lesser restrictions from insur-
    ance providers in your later years.

3. CONSIDER THE OFTEN-NEGLECTED INSURANCE:
    LONG-TERM CARE INSURANCE
    No one knows what the future holds. If we are lucky,
    we will grow old. The truth is that at least 70% of
    Americans who turn age 65 will need some form of
    long-term care. (Administration on Aging, 2014).
    The cost of long-term care depends on the type and
    duration of care needed, the provider chosen, and
    geography. Long-term care insurance is a great op-
    tion for seniors, but it is expensive. In addition, a per-
    son must be in relatively good health to qualify for
    long-term care insurance. If you believe long-term
    care insurance is appropriate for you, experts rec-
    ommend buying in your 40s, since the premium
    continues to rise as you age.

4. IF APPROPRIATE, REVIEW MEDICARE OPTIONS
    The primary choice pertaining to Medicare coverage
    is this: Do you choose Original Medicare (Parts A
    and B) or a Medicare Advantage Plan (Part C)? Use
    the steps that follow to help you decide which option

is best for you. (Refer to the definitions of Parts A, B, C, and D, earlier in this chapter.) As always, when dealing with any federal or state office, be sure to obtain a signed receipt of delivery for any paperwork submitted.

Step 1:

Decide if you want Original Medicare or a Medicare Advantage Plan. Here are some frequently asked questions about Medicare Advantage Plans:

What is a Medicare Advantage Plan (Part C)? Part C includes both Part A (hospital insurance) and Part B (medical insurance).

What entity provides coverage? Private insurance companies approved by Medicare provide Part C coverage.

How do you choose care providers? Most plans require you to use plan doctors, hospitals, and other providers. If you don't, you pay more of or all the costs.

Who pays the premiums? You usually pay a monthly premium in addition to your Part B premium.

Who pays deductibles and coinsurance? You do. You will be financially responsible for any deductibles and coinsurance.

Step 2:

Decide if you want Medicare prescription drug coverage, which is Part D.

If you want prescription drug coverage, and it's offered by your plan, in most cases you must get it through your plan.

In some types of plans that don't offer drug coverage, you can join a Medicare Prescription Drug Plan.

Step 3:

Decide if you want supplemental coverage, which is available only to those who choose Original Medicare.

Step 4:

To receive assistance with Medicare or Medicaid, call the Medicare Help Line, 1-800-MEDICARE (1-800-633-4227), TTY/TDD 1-877-486-2048. In addition to providing assistance surrounding Medicare, this help line will direct you to your state specific Medicaid help line, since every state has different guidelines.

The help line serves all fifty states, the District of Columbia, Puerto Rico, Guam, American Samoa, and the Northern Mariana Islands. You can speak to an English-speaking or Spanish-speaking representative twenty-four hours a day, seven days a week.

CHAPTER 8

DEAL PRODUCTIVELY WITH ANGER AND FRUSTRATION

> *Anger ... it's a paralyzing emotion ... you can't get anything done. People sort of think it's an interesting, passionate, and igniting feeling—I don't think it's any of that—it's helpless ... it's absence of control—and I need all of my skills, all of the control, all of my powers ... and anger doesn't provide any of that—I have no use for it whatsoever.*
>
> ~ Toni Morrison

I'LL NEVER FORGET WHEN THE PHYSICIAN at the pain center promised that the iatrogenic cascade my mother was experiencing would stop with that physician. The doctor made the statement right before she overdosed my mother on a pain medication by failing to adjust the dosage for Mom's renal failure.

In a situation like this, it was difficult not to be angry, and there were so many situations like this. I learned to deal with my anger and frustration in various ways. I began to expect something would go wrong—be it poor communication, redundant testing, or even failure to check patient identification. I coordinated Mom's health

care while constantly assuming the processes or departments involved would fail. Some may say my family
members and I are cynics, but we believe we are realists.
Mom fell victim to so many adverse events that we
would have been foolish to let down our collective guard.

For us, laughter became the best medicine for dealing with the inept health care system. Sure, we got upset
when things went wrong, but our ability to *let go* was
paramount in moving forward and learning to savor
every moment we had with our mother.

Letting go wasn't always easy. It required practice.
Much of my personal anger resulted from lack of care
coordination. I specifically recall Mom's first admission
to the community hospital, where weeks went by without
my seeing Mom's case manager, the person designated
to manage my mother's care. I remember sitting with
my boss, whom I had known for years from a prior position, as I cried and asked how the health care system
could fail so terribly. Although my boss tried, she could
do little to console me; we both knew failure in health
care was a nationwide problem.

My boss and I agreed that the only thing I could do
to prevent errors and help with care coordination was to
be physically present in Mom's room. I was angry that
this was the only solution. The problem wasn't that I
didn't want to be in Mom's room; it was that I shouldn't
have had to coordinate her care. I shouldn't have had to
perform the health care organization's job.

Early on, I learned to utilize the hospital chapel for
respite. I found it was the only place in the entire hospital where I could be alone and others would respect my
privacy. Few people used the chapel. Even when others
were there, the room was always completely quiet. Eve-

ryone was acutely aware that each individual was on a painful journey.

My mother, fortunately, did not remember much of her hospital experience. The human brain has a wonderful way of blocking out many horrific experiences, and patients who are in an ICU for any length of time usually have experiences they're better off forgetting.

By the time Mom was discharged to home, she really had only one glaring reminder of any adverse event, the stage IV bedsore. Her anger about that was continually fresh. There was no letting go for Mom because every time she sat in her wheelchair or every time she lay on her back, she was reminded of things that had gone wrong in the hospital. For some time the bedsore caused her excruciating pain. Every time the rest of the family members saw her grimace in pain, we too, were reminded of all that had gone wrong in the hospital.

In frustration, Mom would say, "Ruthi, do they have any idea how much pain I am in because of the bedsore? They gave me that cheap air mattress to sleep on. I am in pain all day long and all through the night. The pain medication doesn't help at all. If it weren't for the new home care agency, I wouldn't even have this custom wheelchair and new soft cushion. The hospital caused the bedsore and then left me to rot." How could I fail to be angry on Mom's behalf?

Anger is the human response to unmet needs or expectations. When patients enter a hospital, they expect good care and good communication, and they usually expect to leave the hospital in better shape than they were in when admitted. Unfortunately, any deviance in meeting needs or expectations can result in anger. To complicate things, health care providers typically add to this anger by failing to communicate with the patient regarding why expectations were not met.

Providers literally throw fuel on the fire by failing to communicate. This failure can prompt a patient or family to become so angry they consider litigation. They think a lawsuit will make the providers and hospital listen to them. In many cases, they are right.

According to researchers Huntington and Kuhn (2003), the four predominant reasons patients are prompted to file a lawsuit are as follows:

1. Desire to prevent a similar adverse event from happening again
2. Need for an explanation of how and why an injury happened
3. Desire for financial compensation to make up for actual losses, pain, and suffering or to provide future care for the injured patient
4. Desire to hold doctors accountable for their actions

In previous chapters, I discussed how good communication is the foundation of the physician-patient relationship. In addition to yielding better patient outcomes, good communication between a patient and physician has other benefits. Research has shown that patients are less likely to sue physicians they like and trust (Huntington and Kuhn, 2003). Even when a patient has experienced injury as a result of a medical error, the patient is more apt to forgive a physician or the system if the patient and other party have a trusting relationship.

Angry patients can be lawsuits waiting to happen, yet much of their anger can be diffused through communication with their provider, not a lawyer. Patients want to be heard and want their feelings validated. Patients want someone to be accountable for what did or didn't happen. Too many times, no one steps forward. Despite numerous edicts from various agencies (such as the Joint Commission and Institute for Healthcare Improvement), which advocate for full disclosure from hospitals and providers in the case of medical errors, full disclosure has not been fully embraced.

Typically, a patient's or family's anger is directed at the physician because he or she is the most convenient and visible target. One of the worst mistakes a physician can make when dealing with angry patients or families is to avoid them. Although avoidance is an understandable reaction, it is also the surest way to hasten the patient's visit to an attorney's office (Curtis, 2010).

As difficult and unpleasant as it may be, the most effective way to defuse anger is to listen, empathize, and apologize for things that did not turn out the way the patient expected or hoped. Nothing defuses patient anger better than an empathetic health care provider who is willing to acknowledge and discuss the shortcomings of health care, admitting that health care processes and providers need to improve. Studies have shown that, following an error, what patients want from their physicians is an apology and the assurance that what happened to them will not happen to someone else.

Patients are more likely to sue when they believe there is a cover-up of information or when they want more information and the only way they can get it is to file a lawsuit. Litigation seems to be triggered by uncertainty about what happened and how, as well as by unmet expectations (Curtis, 2010).

In my mother's case, with the exception of one ICU nurse who apologized for the bedsore, we never received an official apology from any provider or administrator. In fact—after it was determined that my mother's bedsore was the result of multiple variables, one being the failure of the electronic medical record—the director of nursing defended herself when I learned that the broken process was still not fixed ten months later. "Ruthi," she said, "you know it takes time to fix things."

"How much money will the health system have to pay to a patient's family before they decide to fix it?" I replied, realizing that other patients were still being exposed to the same broken system that gave my mom a stage IV bedsore. I now understood why families sue. I finally got it.

I understood that litigation is often not about money, because no amount of money could take away my mother's pain. No amount of money could bring back the time she lost being heavily medicated for the pain from the bedsore. At times, Mom would require such high doses of narcotics that she couldn't wean from the ventilator. The bedsore affected every aspect of Mom's recovery and life, right up until the day she died. No amount of money would change that. Even so, an apology, or a statement recognizing that the hospital failed her, failed us, and failed as a health care system, would have made a difference. A promise to correct the failed process that caused Mom harm would have made a difference.

The degree of success, whether a doctor or a hospital, isn't always measured by good outcomes. It is measured by what happens after a mistake. We all make mistakes because we're human; it's unavoidable. What is in our control, however, is the way we treat a person and family afterward.

HOSPITAL EXPERIENCES AND POST-TRAUMATIC STRESS

There has been, and continues to be, a significant amount of time and research devoted to post-traumatic stress disorder (PTSD) following an ICU admission. Both patients and their family members typically continue to suffer a range of emotions, including anger, for a long time after an ICU stay. These individuals must make choices about how to respond to lingering intense feelings.

I can only imagine what it is like to be a patient in the ICU. You lie on your back, hearing noises you can't identify, in an environment where bright lights shine twenty-four hours a day. Despite providers' best efforts, this is the stuff horror films are made of. Compound the auditory and visual abnormalities with unfamiliar smells and various medications, and you have a recipe for vivid dreams, hallucinations, and even a syndrome called ICU psychosis.

Most patients in the ICU are on some sort of sedative. If the patient is on a ventilator, providing some kind of medication to alleviate some of the associated anxiety is essential. In addition, ICU patients are likely to be taking narcotics for the treatment of pain. Often such medications induce hallucinations. The recollection of these can be frightening and traumatic and can trigger extreme anxiety days or even months after the patient leaves the ICU (Cartwright, 2012).

Families must be aware of the impact that ICU admission can have on the patient. Although the patient and family may think the worst is over after discharge from the hospital, the effect of the ICU can linger for months. In my mother's case, because of the narcotics she received, she didn't remember much of the six months that she was hospitalized. What Mom did remember was frightening enough for her not to trust hospitals any longer.

Although most research is limited to the patients' experiences, researchers are now beginning to acknowledge the impact that a prolonged ICU stay can have on patients' families. Family members are not immune to post-ICU PTSD. Profound lifestyle disruption—coupled with feelings of helplessness, stress, guilt, and depression—are emotions common to those caring for patients recovering from life-threatening illnesses (Cartwright, 2012).

As an ICU nurse, I watched families of transplant patients sit by their loved ones' bedsides for months. During my mother's ICU stay, my family also had a months-long vigil. Life stops the day your loved one is admitted to the ICU. All chores of daily life seem inconsequential. Once your family member is discharged, it is reasonable to think that life will return to normal, but it isn't so easy.

If you happen to be one of the 100,000 patients (or families of patients) a year who suffer from a medical error, you may suffer from a medically induced trauma (MIT) as a result of the experience. Kenney (2013) defines *medically induced trauma* this way: "Medically Induced Trauma is an unexpected outcome that occurs during medical and/or surgical care that [negatively] affects the emotional well-being [sic] of the patient, family member, and/or clinician(s)."

As a result of MIT, patients and families may feel any of the following:

- Isolated because hospitals in many cases are not set up to provide emotional support beyond the hospital stay
- Mistrustful because the trust between caregiver and patient has been breached
- Vulnerable because the patient typically needs to continue care within the same system that harmed him or her

Patients and families may also feel a mix of emotions following any adverse medical event, including the following:

- Sadness
- Anger
- Isolation
- Guilt
- Shame
- Fear
- Loss
- Desire to connect with others who have had similar experiences
- Gratitude for survival
- Ambivalence
- Protectiveness
- Worry about the health of loved one
- Shock

MIT describes the emotions of my mom and family to a tee. We felt vulnerable because we mistrusted the hospital system that was caring for her. Changing hospitals wasn't the answer, because most of the adverse events were the result of failed processes that occur repeatedly at hospitals all across the country. Rather than change hospitals, we needed to channel our anger into a proactive approach to Mom's care.

My family members made a conscious decision to take control and turn any negative emotions into positive energy directed at change. No one has enough energy to nurse anger and engage in proactive behavior at the same time. We chose to focus all of our energy on improving my mother's quality of life.

Our decision to take my mom home on a ventilator and battle the system to perform home hemodialysis was based on love, not anger. We were angry at the inept U.S. health care system that promotes medical errors through a broken and fragmented infrastructure, but that is not what drove our decision. We decided that, during whatever time my mom had left, she would be as comfortable as possible. As Dorothy in *The Wizard of Oz* says, "There's no place like home." As Glinda, the good witch, points out, Dorothy always had the power to go home. Dorothy just didn't realize it. In a similar way, patients and their families have the power to impact outcomes and patient care by advocating for themselves and speaking out. They always have the power; they just may not realize it.

TURNING ANGER INTO A POSITIVE

When you've been a victim in any experience, including one in health care, you will likely experience some or all of the five stages of grief that Elisabeth Kubler-Ross popularized. These include denial, anger, bargaining, depression, and acceptance (Torrey, 2013).

According to Trisha Torrey (2013), a sixth stage can develop from the process of grief or trauma and its associated anger. A person can emerge with a sense of empowerment and growth. Such a result is called *proactive survivorship*. Torrey notes, "Proactive survivors take a step that goes beyond the five steps of grief to create something good for others. They move from the mindset of being a victim, to the mindset of being a hero to others." Not everyone can move from being the victim to being a proactive survivor, but people can turn anger into a positive force for change.

Proactive survivors are individuals who choose, out of their own painful experience, to champion a cause. Many such individuals find themselves thrust into the limelight as they advocate for change. They start foundations or organizations to raise funds for research, prevent tragedies, remember loved ones who have passed on, or provide support for others. Examples include Christopher Reeve, Michael J. Fox, the sister of Susan G. Komen, Elizabeth Smart, and survivors and families of 9/11.

It never occurred to me that my family's experience in health care could help others until my mother spoke up one day while receiving dialysis at the trauma center. One of the nurses, Jean, was talking to my mom about the nurse's dad, who had just suffered a massive stroke. Jean was in tears, discussing the horrible care her dad was receiving. She was unsure about what the options were, since her dad was a Medicaid patient.

"Ruthi, you need to help her. I feel so bad for her," Mom exclaimed while lying in bed, hooked up to the dialysis machine.

I spoke to Jean that day and touched base with her every few days thereafter, until her father's care and condition improved. Before long, various other acquaintances who heard about the journey I was on with Mom began to approach me for advice about their struggles with health care.

Mom said, "You need to start a business, Ruthi. You need to help other families who don't know how to navigate the hospital system." From this suggestion, my brother, Rick, and I formed the company Eldercare Navigators, LLC, to help others make their way through the complex health care maze. My mother assisted with brainstorming the company name and logo, which is a compass. The company is a natural outgrowth of our decision to deal productively with our own experience of pain and frustration. It is also a fitting way to honor our mother.

What makes some people who have suffered a loss of some kind channel their frustrations and energy into starting a foundation, support group, or company or writing a book? Torrey (2013) answers this way: "Because five steps of grief aren't enough for them. They need that next step—prevention and improvement—to get past their grief and to add to their own quality of life, post-tragedy."

There is definitely truth in this statement because that next step, prevention and improvement, helps to give some meaning to experiences. At least it has for me. Torrey (2013) lists some of the benefits of taking that sixth step to proactive survivorship.

1. PROACTIVE SURVIVORSHIP GIVES YOU CHOICES

   You decide how your loss will influence your life as you move forward. You acknowledge and accept the loss and work with it, not against it. Your choice doesn't make the grief go away or necessarily make it any less intense, but it does give you a sense of control over how you respond to your surroundings and what has happened to you or your loved one.

2. PROACTIVE SURVIVORSHIP BECOMES A CONSTANT BACKDROP TO YOUR ENTIRE LIFE—BUT IN A POSITIVE WAY

   Using your experience and story to help and teach others turns your negative experience into a positive one. This does not mean that you don't acknowledge your horrendous experience. It just means that you now choose to use the experience for good.

3. PROACTIVE SURVIVORSHIP GIVES YOU A STORY TO TELL

   The story allows you to help others along their journey. You use the story to teach and inspire. The telling of a story provides a human connection, a shared experience. Letting others know that you survived and triumphed communicates hope. There is no greater medicine than hope.

4. PROACTIVE SURVIVORSHIP HELPS YOU MOVE BEYOND BLAME

   When you've been a victim in any experience, you can expect to go through some or all of the Kubler-Ross stages—this will eventually help you to cope. But proactive survivorship gives you a reason to celebrate instead of blame. Proactive survivorship, done right, means your experience improves the lives of others.

5. PROACTIVE SURVIVORSHIP GIVES YOU SOMETHING TO DO

If you feel as though you've been victimized but know that, if you had something to do, you would then begin to heal or at least deal with your pain, then proactive survivorship is a solution for you. It doesn't change the difficulty or the outcome, but it gives you a purpose that helps you get past the grief of the original problem or tragedy.

ACTION STEPS FOR YOUR FAMILY

1. BE KIND TO YOURSELF

Often we are kind to others while we push ourselves beyond our own limits. The first step in dealing with anger or frustration is to care for yourself. Well-meaning friends and relatives often tell you to *take care.* But no one will actually tell you *how* to take care of yourself while supporting a loved one or sitting at his or her side at the hospital.

One of the first things I learned was to ask for and accept help. It's important to clearly identify your needs and acknowledge that you can't do it all alone. Make a list of people you know who would be willing to help. Help doesn't necessarily mean caregiving, but every task or chore that is removed from your full plate will give you a few more minutes of you time every day!

2. TAKE SPONTANEOUS AND UNPLANNED BREAKS

If your loved one is in the hospital and needs to have a test, give the nurse your cell number and go sit outside for ten minutes. Once my mother was discharged to home, we used a wireless doorbell for her to call when she needed something. This allowed the caregiver on duty the freedom to be in another room or go outside.

I would take the wireless receiver with me when I went to get the mail. My walk to the mailbox was a mini vacation. Sun, and even rain, can be good for the soul. Exercise of any kind can help to release some of the frustration that caregivers experience. To give myself extra peace of mind on my mini vacations, I also had my Mom wear a Lifeline medical-alert bracelet.

3. PACK A BAG OF YOUR OWN
    Find an attractive cloth bag for essential personal items when you visit the hospital. Keep hand lotion, lip balm, a journal, a novel, or any item that is soothing for you.

4. BE MINDFUL AND MEDITATIVE
    Every hospital has a chapel. Most have a chaplain, at least on call. Consider utilizing available resources for prayer or reflection. Pick up a book on mindfulness meditation. Carry a book on mindfulness with you and read a passage or two when you have a few minutes. Use a journal to jot down your thoughts and feelings.

Being mindful reminds us to have gratitude for even the small mundane things—after all, they can go away in a flash. When caring for your loved one, be mindful of how he or she feels, smells, talks, laughs, etc. Appreciate the beauty of it all. The memories you make in doing so can be conjured up at a moment's notice . . . forever. Seize the opportunity to be present in the moment. Refuse to let anger rob you of valuable time.

5. **NOURISH YOUR BODY WITH HEALTHY FOOD**

It is all too easy to rely on junk food and vending machines. Avoid using alcohol or drugs (including caffeine) to get through the day. These will only complicate things and add to the anger and frustration. Eating healthy food will give you the physical and mental stamina to deal with whatever is thrown your way during the day. Ultimately, it will help you to deal with adversity more effectively.

After my mother was discharged to home, I didn't want to have to spend precious time grocery shopping. I placed an ad on Craigslist for a grocery shopper (I had 30 people apply) and hired a woman for $10/hour. It was the best money I ever spent. I was able to make out a list of healthy food for Mom and me and eliminate the dreaded chore of grocery shopping.

6. **SLEEP WHENEVER YOU CAN**

Many of us struggle with sleep even without a life crisis. If you have an unexpected two-hour break in the middle of an afternoon, take a nap and refuse to feel guilty about it. Sleep, like healthy food, helps all of us handle adversity better. In addition to sleep, keep up with your own health needs. Don't skip annual medical screenings or allow yourself to run out of prescription medicine. If you do not take care of yourself, you can't do a good job of caring for your loved one.

At one point while caring for my mother at home, she said, "Is all you ever do sleep?" Of course, Mom didn't realize I was often up at night while she was sleeping or that the doctor called my house at 6 every morning while she was hospitalized. I slept when I had the opportunity and didn't feel the need to explain myself.

7. LAUGH, LAUGH, LAUGH

We all know the power of a good belly laugh! Try to see the humor in life. Before Mom's illness, I watched certain dramas and medical shows on TV. I also read various nursing journals in the evenings. During Mom's illness, I watched sitcoms and read gossip magazines. No news, no medical shows or dramas, and no additional misery were permitted in my life. On my bathroom mirror, I wrote in lipstick "One Day at a Time." This was my mantra.

8. AVOID HARD AND FAST PLANS

Purchasing tickets for concerts or signing up to take a class and then being unable to attend can add to your frustration. You are often better off using any free time to take a walk, shop, or even nap. Time becomes ever so precious. Learn to use it wisely.

9. CONSIDER COUNSELING

Many counselors specialize in anger, the stress of caregiving, and grief. If you need help in getting through a stressful time in life, you are not weak or unusual. Think about what you need or want. Do you just want to talk to someone? Maybe a therapist or support group is what you need. If you think you might need medications, consult your PCP or a psychiatrist.

Many caregivers have trouble sleeping or find themselves battling anxiety. Don't be ashamed or embarrassed to ask your doctor for medications to help with sleep or anxiety problems. If your loved one is hospitalized and you are caring for him or her far from where you live, ask a nurse or doctor to refer you to the appropriate professional near the hospital. Health care providers and social workers are used to assisting out-of-town visitors with their health care needs.

Regardless of your location, if you are having difficulty coping with the anger or frustration of being a patient or caregiver, reach out to a mental health professional. For those caregivers unable to leave the home but in need of support, many online support groups are available. Support groups for caregivers, relating to specific diseases, are constantly being added to the online community. For a list of current online support communities, type "online caregiver support group" into your digital search engine.

CHAPTER 9

SAY GOOD BYE AS YOUR LOVED ONE AND FAMILY CHOOSE

> *Ever has it been that love knows not its own depth until the hour of separation.*
>
> ~ Kahlil Gibran

IN JULY 2012, AFTER RECEIVING IV antibiotics at home for three MONTHS because of unrelenting pneumonia, Mom was hospitalized for the first time in fifteen months. The decision to have her admitted was a difficult one. Mom agreed to the decision despite all the previous difficulties. She had had fifteen months of freedom and some control in her life, but her increased difficulty in breathing while on the ventilator forced us to call an ambulance.

My mother was in the Emergency Department at the familiar community hospital for only thirty minutes before she regretted coming to the hospital. "Ruthi, I can't breathe. This ventilator isn't helping at all. I need suctioned. Suction me!" she mouthed since the tracheostomy and ventilator prevented audible words.

"I can't, Mom. We're at the hospital, and they have to do it. I'm not allowed. The nurse said she called the respiratory therapist to suction you."

"I'm going to die right here in the Emergency De-partment. Why can't the nurse suction me? I can't breathe!" Mom continued to mouth words as her respira-tory rate increased to a worrisome forty breaths per minute.

Just then, Dr. Quarterson entered the room. He looked at the monitor and listened to my mother's lungs, "Your oxygen saturation number is good at 95%."

"I don't care what it is," she said, "I can't breathe. I need suctioned."

"A respiratory therapist will be here shortly. Maybe they need to adjust your ventilator settings since we switched you from your home vent to the hospital vent. They'll check it," Dr. Quarterson said as he patted my mom's arm and walked out of the room.

Mom's response was, "Ruthi, I want to go home. I'd rather die at home. Get me out of here. Why did I come here if they won't help me? I'll be dead before I ever come back to the hospital again."

A respiratory therapist did come and adjust the vent, and my mother's breathing improved, but the emotional damage was done. This experience was the deciding one; Mom vowed she was finished with hospitals. This would be her last hospital visit.

My mother was admitted to the ICU that day and started on new IV antibiotics. Within twenty-four hours, she was feeling better and requesting food and her iPad. She also told her PCP, Dr. Farrell, she was ready to leave. Despite the recommendation that she stay in the hospital until the specific type of bacteria causing her pneumonia was identified, Dr. Farrell agreed to let her go home the following day. He couldn't help but side with my mother as he watched her sitting in a chair in the ICU, on the ventilator and eating an egg-salad sandwich, clam chowder, and peach pie with ice cream. Mom ate while playing Scrabble on her iPad and mouthing words to her nurse to heat up her pie so the vanilla ice cream would melt a bit. No one quite knew what to do with Mom at this point. Staff members weren't used to having an 83-year-old vent patient like her in the ICU. Mom was nothing if not resilient.

When Mom was discharged on July 16, we had no idea that she would die exactly one month later. She was full of life for the 2½ weeks following discharge, savoring every moment at home. Mom then had an unanticipated mental status change and took a turn for the worse. She was in a confused state, consistent with that of an elderly woman with a severe infection. The best efforts of all of her doctors, as well as lab tests and a new antibiotic, weren't enough. This was the turning point for our family.

There comes a time when—despite your own and your family's wishes, beliefs, or hope—death stares you in the face. I had seen it in my mother's eyes when it was time to let my dad go. I had seen it with countless transplant-recipient families, and I was now seeing it in the eyes of my siblings.

A defining moment comes when you, as a family member, realize you are no longer prolonging a loved one's life but prolonging your loved one's dying process. I have learned that no one can tell you when that time is; it is a point that you must reach on your own.

The decision to let go is usually made after endless hours at your loved one's bedside, recognizing the pain and suffering your loved one has endured. I have watched countless doctors and nurses attempt to convey the need to make a decision to a family, but the advice is usually offered in vain. The timing is personal to each family.

When my mother's mental status changed, she was on a ventilator at night and receiving home hemodialysis. The ventilator allowed her to rest at night, which ultimately strengthened her enough to allow her to breathe on her own without a vent during the day. Dialysis, however, was another issue. Without the dialysis that cleaned Mom's blood of fatal toxins, she would die. After consultation with Dr. Farrell, we decided to stop dialysis and keep my mother as comfortable as possible. With our consent, Dr. Farrell placed the order for hospice to come to the house and assist the family with end-of-life care for my mother.

END-OF-LIFE OPTIONS

Families can make various choices at the end of life. Different agencies can assist with the final days, depending upon the needs and wants of the patient and family. Most of the services can be provided in almost any setting, such as a hospital, nursing home, assisted living facility, or home environment. Both hospice and palliative care are available to provide end-of-life care. The major differences between the two involve the expected length of time until death and whether curative treatment is still being provided. In both cases, you can expect the services listed below. Typically, insurance will cover most or all of the services.

The word *palliative* is defined as "providing relief." Although there is a distinct difference between palliative and hospice care, there is also a relationship between the two. By definition, palliative care focuses on relieving symptoms and pain related to chronic illnesses, such as cancer, cardiac disease, respiratory disease, kidney failure, Alzheimer's and other dementias, AIDS, and amyotrophic lateral sclerosis (ALS) and other neurological diseases.

Hospice provides relief and additional support when a cure is no longer an option. Palliative care for the dying is called hospice care. Both provide whole-person and family support as well as symptom relief.

The hospice concept traveled to the United States from London, where the philosophy and principles (described below) were introduced in the 1970s. The approach gained acceptance, and Medicare began covering its costs in 1982.

Hospice is actually a philosophy, involving a care plan and sometimes even a facility. Hospice care provides comfort and support to terminally ill patients and their families. Hospice acknowledges death as a natural occurrence and the inevitable conclusion of life. The goal of hospice is to provide pain control and comfort to the patient, which ultimately provides a better quality of life in the final stages of terminal illness.

Years ago, a hospice was a place that dying patients went to die. Although this is still an option for those who require complicated care or who do not have family or friends who can assist, many patients opt for hospice care at home. Patients also receive hospice care in nursing homes, residential facilities, and acute-care hospitals. Not surprisingly, with the growth of the elderly population, there has been a steady increase in hospice care provided in nursing homes over the last fifteen years.

To be admitted to hospice care, the patient's physician must write an order indicating that treatment options for a specific illness have been exhausted, the patient's life expectancy is six months or fewer, and the time to focus on end-of-life care has come. Even with hospice, a patient may still receive medical treatment for any unrelated illnesses that are not strictly symptoms of the terminal illness.

The fundamental principle of hospice is holistic care. The whole person—including body, mind, and spirit—is treated.

According to the National Hospice and Palliative Care Organization (2012), the basic tenets of hospice care include the following:

- Management of pain associated with the terminal illness
- Support for the emotional, spiritual, and social needs of patients and families
- Help that allows individual patients to maintain dignity and some control over the manner in which they die

In addition, the interdisciplinary hospice team:

- Provides needed drugs, medical supplies, and equipment
- Instructs the family how to care for the patient
- Delivers special services like speech and physical therapy
- Makes short-term inpatient care available when pain or symptoms become too difficult to treat at home or the caregiver needs respite
- Provides bereavement care and counseling to surviving family and friends

Most patients receive care under one of the following four levels of hospice care:

Level 1:   Routine home care
           Patient receives hospice care at the place of residence.

Level 2:   Continuous home care
           Patient receives hospice care consisting primarily of licensed nursing care on a continuous basis at home.

Level 3:   General inpatient care
           Patient receives general inpatient care, in an inpatient facility, for pain control or acute or complex symptom management that cannot be managed in other settings.

Level 4:   Inpatient respite care
           Patient receives care in an approved facility on a short-term basis to provide respite for the caregiver.

MAJOR DIFFERENCES BETWEEN PALLIATIVE AND HOSPICE CARE

- Palliative care can be used at any stage of illness—not just the advanced stages. Treatments are not limited with palliative care and can range from conservative to aggressive or curative.
- Hospice treatment is limited, and its focus is on relief of symptoms. The goal is no longer to cure but to promote comfort.
- Palliative care can be considered at any time during the course of a chronic illness.

- With hospice care, Medicare requires that a physician certify a patient's condition as terminal. The physician must certify that a patient's life expectancy is six months or fewer. Although a physician's referral is needed for palliative care, the patient does not need to be declared terminal; there can still be hope for a cure.

- Both palliative and hospice care can be delivered at any location.

- Palliative care includes specialists, non-physician clinicians, social workers, chaplains, pharmacists, and nutritionists.

- Hospice care includes physicians, nurses, social workers, spiritual caregivers, bereavement specialists, and volunteers.

Because of the increasingly older population in the United States and the chronic diseases that often plague this group, palliative care is a rapidly growing field. Many specialists—such as cardiologists, pulmonologists, nephrologists, and other doctors who care for patients with chronic diseases—are familiar with providing a referral for palliative care services. Have a conversation with your doctor to discuss the options.

For the same reasons, hospice is also a rapidly growing field. To have a conversation about hospice, contact your PCP.

Regardless of the final path you choose for yourself or your loved one, you will never know how long it will actually take until death comes. Predicting the time of death is even more difficult than predicting the time of birth. Professionals can make an educated guess, but at the end of the day, it is an educated guess and nothing more.

MOM AS AN OUTLIER

Nothing about my mother's illness and recovery was easy. In fact, my mother was an outlier along every step of the way. For this reason, we had to battle the insurance company, Medicare, Medicaid, and countless other entities. When it came time for Mom to die, it shouldn't have come as a surprise to us that Mom was considered an outlier then as well.

When my mother had mental status changes of an unknown origin, Dr. Farrell wrote an order for hospice services with the diagnosis of end-stage renal failure. We knew this meant we would no longer dialyze my mother Because of the buildup of toxins in her blood, she would slowly succumb to her death.

For hospice services, we chose the same faith-based home care agency that had provided my mother with the customized wheelchair and cushion. This agency had delivered holistic care from the moment a staff member entered our home. This agency had a hospice division, and we were confident this agency could effectively guide us through Mom's final days and hours.

Dr. Farrell's office nurse contacted the agency for hospice services for Mom at 9:30 a.m. At 2 p.m., when the nurse, Jenna, came to admit Mom to hospice services, my mother was in bed, resting quietly on the ventilator with her eyes closed.

After asking me multiple questions and finding Mom's past history from prior home care visits in her computer, Jenna went into Mom's room to assess her.

She deferred taking vital signs, per my request, as I did not want my mother disturbed to obtain numbers that were irrelevant at this point. Jenna remarked about the ventilator, saying that my mother looked comfortable and appeared to be breathing easily. I explained to Jenna that my mother could breathe easily on her own; Mom used the ventilator to help her rest while sleeping.

Jenna finished her visit by explaining the services hospice offered for Mom and describing the bereavement services that would be offered to my family for the next year. I was thankful for hospice because I truly wanted to assume the role of the daughter at this point. Although I knew that I would help to make Mom comfortable in her final days, I was looking to hospice to guide the process and provide support not only to my mother, but also to my family and me.

Jenna reviewed the list of medications that had been ordered for Mom, carefully explaining what each one was for and when to give it. The total process took about 2½ hours. I remember feeling frustrated because I would rather have spent the time with my mother.

The medications arrived within the hour, and my family and I began administering them as ordered. We removed any unneeded medical equipment from Mom's room and placed it on the huge front porch. I was placing additional chairs in my mom's room when the telephone rang.

"Ruth, this is the hospice administrator, Debbie. I'm sorry to tell you this, but we can't provide care to your mother."

Startled, I asked, "What do you mean?"

"We didn't know your mother was on a ventilator. I just realized it now, when I read the assessment form."

"How could you not know? Your agency took care of her before, and you knew she was on a vent at night. Plus, the nurse was just in her room while she was on the ventilator. Your nurse didn't say anything."

"Well, Jenna is new. And I don't know why we didn't catch it, but we didn't realize that she was on a ventilator. I called Dr. Farrell about this issue, and he told me that you are a nurse. He will write an order for the medications to make your mother comfortable. We are not permitted to admit anyone to hospice who is on a ventilator."

I sat in disbelief. "My mother only uses the vent to rest while sleeping. She can breathe on her own. The ventilator is not a curative treatment. We only use the ventilator to make her comfortable. The dialysis was keeping Mom alive, and we have stopped dialysis. I don't understand why you will not provide services."

"It's our policy. We've always done it this way. I'm sorry," the administrator said in a whisper.

It's our policy. . . . It's our rule. . . . We've always done it this way. . . . These phrases created unreasonable obstacles right to the very end.

Even at the very end, my mother would be an outlier. She would not fit into the mold that the U.S. health system created. Once again, we were forced to work around an inept system to deliver the care that my mother needed and deserved. Although I was disappointed with the failure of a system to provide end-of-life care, my family and I were privileged to provide such sacred care during Mom's final days.

Once again, my family members rallied to provide the level of care we believed to be in Mom's best interest.

Kathy and Catie, my sister and my niece, became the primary caregivers from 7 p.m. to 7 a.m. Catie assessed her grandmother throughout the night for any discomfort and medicated her accordingly. My sister-in-law, Debbie, and I provided care throughout the day. My brothers were at Mom's bedside as well, ensuring there was always at least one person with her twenty-four hours a day. Mom also received visits from her sisters, in-laws, nieces, and nephews.

Throughout the next week, we prepared for the funeral and made a video and numerous photo collages of Mom's life. We found it cathartic as we realized that Mom was smiling in every picture. We reflected on her 83 years of life and remarked that we could only wish we would all be so lucky to live a life as full as Mom's.

My mother died a peaceful death on August 16, 2012, surrounded by her family, ten days after we stopped dialysis. We thought it fitting that her six children were her pallbearers. She brought us into this world, and it was only natural that we accompanied her out.

ACTION STEPS FOR YOUR FAMILY

1. TALK ABOUT THE FUTURE WITH YOUR PCP
    If you or your loved one has a chronic disease that is progressing, initiate a discussion with your PCP. Some physicians may feel uncomfortable starting this conversation, especially if the patient has had a long-term relationship with the doctor. The doctor might be afraid the patient will think that he or she is giving up and not providing optimal care.

Although palliative care can benefit many patients, many patients never take advantage of the services. Palliative care can provide you or your loved one a better quality of life, often within the confines of your own home.

2. DECIDE WHERE TO SPEND FINAL DAYS

If you or your loved one is progressing along a chronic disease continuum, there may be a point at which you decide not to re-enter a hospital. Consider the questions that follow for yourself or with your loved one: If you do enter a hospital, you might ask yourself why you are returning there. Are you seeking new treatment or relief of symptoms? Is it possible for you to receive the same care at home? If you are unable to receive the care at home and do not wish to re-enter the hospital, discuss alternatives with your doctor.

3. INVESTIGATE HOSPICE

My family's experience with hospice was less than ideal, because my mother did not fit the standard criteria for hospice. Many patients and families who utilize hospice services are very pleased with the care provided. In addition, patients who access palliative care also report a better quality of life because the symptoms of their disease are better controlled.

Because of the emotional toll that the end of life places on a patient and family, expecting the family to investigate several facilities or organizations before making a decision may be unrealistic. Most times, relying on the recommendation of a family member, friend, or PCP, in regard to the choice of a hospice provider, is appropriate

4. **COMMUNICATE WISHES AT EVERY STEP**

   I've mentioned earlier how important it is to have discussions about your own and your loved one's wishes. However unpleasant the discussions may be at the time, they make future decision-making much easier and allow the wishes of the dying to be honored. In addition, be sure you or your loved one designates the power of attorney and a health care surrogate and has a living will, to ensure that final wishes are honored.

   As the end of life approaches, take cues from your loved one. Don't assume your loved one does not want to talk about end-of-life issues and wishes.

5. **DON'T UNDERESTIMATE YOUR PERSONAL RESOURCES**

   In regard to hospice care, patients and families can decide if the services are right for them and what hospice environment is most appropriate. Many individuals choose to die at home. This can be arranged through hospice with the help of family or friends. Families often surprise themselves at what caregiving tasks they can accomplish. I have never met a family member who wasn't grateful for the opportunity to care for his or her loved one at the end of that person's life.

6. **DO YOUR BEST TO HONOR WISHES**

   If your loved one can no longer communicate wishes, think about what he or she would want. If your loved one has expressed the desire to be an organ or tissue donor, let his or her physician know. Depending on the situation, this may still be possible.

   Various cultures and religions have specific rituals that must be followed during and after a death. Call your priest, minister, rabbi, or spiritual leader earlier rather than later. If your loved one will pass in a hospital or other nursing facility, make the facility aware of your needs. Health care providers can accommodate any religious or cultural custom.

7. INFORM FAMILY MEMBERS WHO MAY WANT TO SAY GOOD-BYE
   Many families fear calling others too early to say the final good-bye to a dying person. This struggle is unnecessary. If your loved one lives for a few weeks or months after others have said their good-byes, be thankful. Again, no one knows when the end will come for sure; all you can do is make an educated guess.

8. ARRANGE FOR YOUR FINAL GOOD-BYE
   It is okay and even advisable to contact the funeral home before your loved one passes. It is okay to make your loved one aware of your plans. He or she may have specific wishes for the funeral, religious service, memorial, or burial. Follow your loved one's cues. If funeral arrangements are not complete at the time of death, take someone with you to the funeral home. It is easy to spend a lot of money when you are grieving and emotionally exhausted.

9. MAKE THE TIME YOU HAVE COUNT
   Above all, be present with your loved one. No one should die alone if it can be prevented. Let your loved one feel your love. Provide gentle touch, massage, comforting words, and music, as appropriate.

As your loved one moves toward the end of life, come together as a family in a way that works for you. Look at photo albums, tell stories, play music, laugh and cry together. Fill this special time in ways that heal and bless your unique family.

10. Use the Broad Range of Services Available for the Whole Family

Each family member will process grief in his or her own way. Remember to call upon hospice, your spiritual resources, social resources, and professional help as needed. Support each other by talking about your loved one, telling his or her story, planting a memorial, and participating in proactive survivorship in memory of your loved one.

CHAPTER 10

ONE YEAR LATER

> *Whoever survives a test, whatever it may be,*
> *must tell the story. That is his duty.*
> ~ Elie Wiesel

T HE FIRST YEAR AFTER ANY LOSS is the most difficult. It
is a year full of change and adjustment. Life doesn't
go back to *normal*, but you do find a *new normal*. My
family and I find solace in the wonderful memories we
have of my mother, and many of those memories were
made during the last few years of her life, when Mom
was ill. I think my mother would be proud of the progress we've made during the first year after her death.

Immediately following her passing, my goal was to
donate all of Mom's medical supplies. I thought it would
be easy to donate medical supplies, but because of her
complex medical issues we had supplies that most organizations weren't used to accepting. Those that would
accept the supplies requested that we bring the supplies
to them. This was difficult, since we had a basement full
of supplies, including 60 cases of dialysis solution.

After I searched for six weeks, Brother's Brother
Foundation was the organization that sent a team of
men, along with a large truck, to the house and loaded
every supply. Later that evening, they sent the truck to

the East Coast, where the contents were loaded on a ship bound for Haiti. We donated some equipment we had purchased to Mom's physical therapist. We donated the equipment with one caveat: It had to go to a patient who otherwise could not afford it. When that patient was done with the equipment, he or she had to donate it to another. No one was permitted to make money from our donation. Mom would have been proud that she was able to help others even after her death.

Of course, not everything always goes smoothly after the death of a loved one. Opening up the estate of your family member, dealing with Medicaid issues, and notifying vendors and insurers is not easy. I didn't realize how long it would take to notify everyone involved in Mom's care.

In fact, despite the fact that all parties (doctors, medical equipment companies, and insurance company) were notified, I received a call every Sunday evening at 6:30 from the hospital system. I could set my watch by the automated call. Its purpose was to find out how the patient (my mother) was doing with her respiratory equipment. You were to press 1 if everything was okay, etc. This call persisted for eight months after Mom's death. I attempted to call the number back, but all I got was another automated menu. At first, I was angry at the insensitivity, but I then began to laugh. Even after Mom's death, the broken health care system prevailed.

Being reminded of the broken health care system made it easier for my brother and me to forge ahead with our company, Eldercare Navigators, LLC. Delving into meaningful work, like helping others navigate the complex health and legal system, is gratifying. This is especially true for us with our business, because we both know how stressful and emotionally exhausting the journey can be for a patient and family.

Since the inception of our company, I have encountered health care providers—in fact, too many to count—who have offered to work for us or even volunteer to help seniors navigate the system. Health care providers know the system is broken, and most truly are committed to helping patients receive the best possible care.

In a prior chapter, I mentioned TARP, the Tarantine Assistance Recovery Plan, which was our label for the collaborative effort we put forth in my mother's recovery. TARP still exists, but its meaning has changed to the Tarantine Annual Reunion Plan.

We all decided to rent a house in the Outer Banks in August of the year following Mom's death. Ironically, the week that most family members were available was the week surrounding the anniversary of her death. Although the anniversary was certainly a sad occasion, being together while sharing memories and making new ones helped to ease the pain. We laughed a lot that week, all of us realizing how blessed we are to have so many wonderful memories. In addition, we all realized how blessed we were to be able to do what we did for our mother during the last few years of her life.

SURVIVING

The Oxford Dictionary of English (2013) defines the word *survival* as "the state or fact of continuing to live or exist, typically in spite of an accident, ordeal, or difficult circumstances." Although I agree with this definition, I believe that survival is so much more.

Survival involves taking control of your life and being proactive with the decisions. Surviving a journey through the U.S. health care system involves more than getting out alive. Sometimes survival, as I define it, means holding on to your own dignity and dying on your own terms.

True survival is measured not only by continuance of life, but also by the patient's or family's satisfaction with the overall experience. Even though a patient might be discharged from a hospital, the experience may have been a horrific one for the patient and family. Emotional scars left on patients and families can have profound lifelong effects.

Health care initiatives are helping to bring concern for the satisfaction of patients back into the system, and the days of having blind faith in health care are long gone. Self-determination, the process by which a person controls his or her own life, is paramount to surviving health care, both physically and mentally.

Reflecting on my mother's journey, I realize that she was a true survivor. Yes, she physically survived the surgeries, treatments, and hospitalizations. More important, she mentally survived because she adjusted her expectations based on her changing health. When her body threw her a curve ball, she accepted it and made the best out of the situation. She survived her long journey because she was able to flex her expectations and redefine *quality of life* based on the physical limitations presented to her. My mother always said, "God doesn't give you more than you can handle." I'm not so sure about this, but she was, and that's all that mattered.

In my nursing career, I have heard many of my peers make comments such as, "I would *never* want to live like that," or "I would *never* have a transplant" or be on a ventilator, etc. Never say *never* because life doesn't always work the way you hope it will. My mother used to say, "Just because I'm 82 doesn't mean I don't want to be 83!" We all want more time, and most of us will go to great lengths to get it.

You can learn to be a survivor! Whether you are a patient or family member, the key points in this book will help you on your health care journey:

- If you are a patient, make a conscious decision about how you want to live out your life and convey your wishes to your family members.

- Be present. Be involved. Demand patient-centered care. Remember the adage: Nothing about me without me.

- Advocate for *your* definition of *quality of life.* Your definition is the *only* one that matters.

- Create a notebook to keep records. Be fastidious about this because, in many cases, you'll be the only one with the complete picture.

- Ask for help and accept help. A family member or friend does not have to provide direct care to make your load lighter. People can help with grocery shopping, childcare, housekeeping, etc. Every task matters.

- Learn to cooperate with health care providers to get the care that you want. If you are the pa-tient, you are the most important team mem-ber in your care.

- Acknowledge the broken health care system. Accept that the system is not perfect, and take steps to mitigate the impact of the broken system on your health.

- Be cautious when moving along the care continuum (hospital to nursing home, etc.). Do not let hospitals rush you to make a specific move. You have the right to choose a facility. Also, remember that things often fall through the cracks when care is transferred from one facility to the next. Have all of your medical records to help prevent issues.

- Learn to navigate within your health insurance/Medicare/Medicaid maze. Don't be afraid to challenge the system. Refuse to accept *We've always done it this way* as an answer.

- Utilize available resources. Consult with social workers, case managers, Area Agency on Aging, etc.

- Learn to deal productively with any anger over the failed health care system.

- Know that palliative care and hospice may be options.

We can all survive the journey through the U.S. health care system by employing the fundamental actions that will help us to take and maintain control of our lives. Remember, life can change on a dime. Most of us will find ourselves on a journey through the health care system at some point in our lifetime. Be prepared for your journey. In the meantime, remember to stop and smell the roses along the way.

APPENDIX A: THE PATIENT'S BILL OF RIGHTS

There's no one single patient's bill of rights. As health care has changed, various types of bills of rights have been written. While new rights are taking effect as the result of the Patient Protection and Affordable Care Act of 2010 (see Chapter 7), older bills of rights still apply. The points that follow summarize the Consumer Bill of Rights and Responsibilities that the U.S. Advisory Commission on Consumer Protection and Quality in the Health Care Industry adopted in 1998 (American Cancer Society, 2013).

This bill of rights addresses eight key areas:

1. INFORMATION FOR PATIENTS
    You have the right to accurate and easily understood information about your health plan, health care professionals, and health care facilities.

2. CHOICE OF PROVIDERS AND PLANS
    You have the right to choose health care providers who can give you high-quality health care when you need it.

3. ACCESS TO EMERGENCY SERVICES
    If you have severe pain, an injury, or sudden illness that makes you believe your health is in danger, you have the right to be screened and stabilized using emergency services. You should be able to use these services whenever and wherever you need them,

even if they're out of your network, without needing to wait for authorization and without any financial penalty.

4.   TAKING PART IN TREATMENT DECISIONS

You have the right to know your treatment options and take part in decisions about your care. You have the right to ask about the pros and cons of any treatment, including no treatment at all. As long as you are able to make sound decisions, you have the right to refuse any test or treatment, even if it means you might have a bad health outcome as a result. Legally, you have the right to choose who can speak for you if you cannot make your own decisions.

5.   RESPECT AND NONDISCRIMINATION

You have a right to considerate, respectful care from your doctors, health plan representatives, and other health care providers—care that does not discriminate against you based on race, ethnicity, national origin, religion, sex, age, mental or physical disability, sexual orientation, genetic information, or source of payment.

6.   CONFIDENTIALITY (PRIVACY) OF HEALTH INFORMATION

You have the right to talk privately with health care providers and have your health care information protected. In addition, you have the right to read and copy your own medical record. You have the right to ask that your doctor change your record if it's not correct, relevant, or complete.

7.   COMPLAINTS AND APPEALS

You have the right to a fair, fast, and objective review of any complaint you have against your health plan, doctors, hospitals, or other health care personnel.

This includes complaints about waiting times, operating hours, the actions of health care personnel, and the adequacy of health care facilities.

8. CONSUMER RESPONSIBILITIES

In a health care system that protects consumers' and patients' rights, consumers and patients should expect to take on some responsibilities. For instance, patients must tell their health care providers about any medicines they are taking and about health conditions and medical or surgical problems in the past or present. Patients must ask questions or request further information from health care providers if they do not completely understand health information and instructions.

OTHER BILLS OF RIGHTS

The 1998 Consumer Bill of Rights and Responsibilities focuses on health insurance plans, but there are many other bills of rights, each with a different focal point. Focuses include rights related to

1. People in hospitals
   - High-quality hospital care
   - A clean and safe environment
   - Patient involvement in care
   - Privacy protection
   - Help when leaving the hospital
   - Help with billing claims
2. Mental health
3. Hospice care

Certain U.S. states have their own bills of rights for patients. Insurance plans sometimes have lists that summarize the rights of subscribers. The American Hospital Association (2013), in a booklet called *The Patient Care Partnership,* lists patients' rights along with patients' responsibilities. This booklet can help a caregiver or patient be a more active partner in hospital-provided health care. The booklet is available at http://www.aha.org; search "patient care partnership."

Appendix B: Serious Reportable Events

Serious reportable events were formerly known as never events.

The term *never event* was first introduced in 2001 by Ken Kizer, MD, former CEO of the National Quality Forum (NQF). Never events are medical errors that should never happen. In 2002, twenty-seven never events were listed by NQF, and the list continues to expand. The most recent revision, 2011, lists 29 events grouped into six categories: surgical, product or device, patient protection, care management, environmental, radiologic, and criminal (National Quality Health Forum, 2011).

National Quality Forum's Health Care Never Events (2011 Revision)

Surgical Events
- Surgery or other invasive procedure performed on the wrong body part
- Surgery or other invasive procedure performed on the wrong patient
- Wrong surgical or other invasive procedure performed on a patient
- Unintended retention of a foreign object in a patient after surgery or other procedure

- Intraoperative or immediately postoperative or postprocedure death in an American Society of Anesthesiologists Class I patient

PRODUCT OR DEVICE EVENTS

- Patient death or serious injury associated with the use of contaminated drugs, devices, or biologics provided by the health care setting
- Patient death or serious injury associated with the use or function of a device in patient care, in which the device is used for functions other than as intended
- Patient death or serious injury associated with intravascular air embolism that occurs while being cared for in a health care setting

PATIENT PROTECTION EVENTS

- Discharge or release of a patient/resident of any age, who is unable to make decisions, to other than an authorized person
- Patient death or serious disability associated with patient elopement (disappearance)
- Patient suicide, attempted suicide, or self-harm resulting in serious disability, while being cared for in a health care facility

CARE MANAGEMENT EVENTS

- Patient death or serious injury associated with a medication error (e.g., errors involving the wrong drug, wrong dose, wrong patient, wrong time, wrong rate, wrong preparation, or wrong route of administration)
- Patient death or serious injury associated with unsafe administration of blood products

- Maternal death or serious injury associated with labor or delivery in a low-risk pregnancy while being cared for in a health care setting
- Death or serious injury of a neonate associated with labor or delivery in a low-risk pregnancy
- Artificial insemination with the wrong donor sperm or wrong egg
- Patient death or serious injury associated with a fall while being cared for in a health care setting
- Any stage 3, stage 4, or unstageable pressure ulcers acquired after admission/presentation to a health care facility
- Patient death or serious disability resulting from the irretrievable loss of an irreplaceable biological specimen
- Patient death or serious injury resulting from failure to follow up or communicate laboratory, pathology, or radiology test results

ENVIRONMENTAL EVENTS
- Patient or staff death or serious disability associated with an electric shock in the course of a patient care process in a health care setting
- Any incident in which a line designated for oxygen or other gas to be delivered to a patient contains no gas, the wrong gas, or is contaminated by toxic substances
- Patient or staff death or serious injury associated with a burn incurred from any source in the course of a patient care process in a health care setting

- Patient death or serious injury associated with the use of restraints or bedrails while being cared for in a health care setting

RADIOLOGIC EVENTS

- Death or serious injury of a patient or staff associated with introduction of a metallic object into the MRI area

CRIMINAL EVENTS

- Any instance of care ordered by or provided by someone impersonating a physician, nurse, pharmacist, or other licensed health care provider
- Abduction of a patient/resident of any age
- Sexual abuse/assault on a patient within or on the grounds of a health care setting
- Death or significant injury of a patient or staff member resulting from a physical assault (i.e., battery) that occurs within or on the grounds of a health care setting

REFERENCES AND KEY SOURCES

Administration on Aging, U.S. Department of Health and
    Human Services. (2013). Long-term care ombudsman
    program. Retrieved from http://www.aoa.gov/
    aoa_programs/elder_rights/Ombudsman/

Administration on Aging, U.S. Department of Health and
    Human Services. (2014). Who needs care? Retrieved
    from http://longtermcare.gov/the-basics/who-needs-care/

Agency for Healthcare Research and Quality, U.S. Depart-
    ment of Health & Human Services. (2012). Never
    events. Retrieved from http://www.psnet.ahrq.gov/
    primer.aspx?primerID=3

Agency for Healthcare Research and Quality, U.S. Depart-
    ment of Health & Human Services. (2014). Making sure
    your surgery is safe. Retrieved from
    http://www.ahrq.gov/patients-consumers/diagnosis-
    treatment/surgery/index.html

Aging with Dignity. (2013). Five wishes. Retrieved from
    http://www.agingwithdignity.org/five-wishes.php

American Association of Colleges of Nursing. (2013). End-of-
    life nursing education consortium fact sheet. Retrieved
    from http://www.aacn.nche.edu/elnec/FactSheet.pdf

American Cancer Society. (2013). Patient's Bill of Rights. Retrieved from http://www.cancer.org/treatment/ findingandpayingfortreatment/understanding financialandlegalmatters/patients-bill-of-rights

American Hospital Association. (2013). The patient care partnership. Retrieved from http://www.aha.org/advocacy-issues/communicatingpts/pt-care-partnership.shtml

American Thoracic Society. (2013). Code status. Retrieved from http://www.thoracic.org/clinical/critical-care/patient-information/code-status.php

Berwick, D. (2004). *Escape fire: Designs for the future of health care.* San Francisco: Jossey-Bass.

Blumberg, A., & Davidson, A. (Narrators). (2009, October 22). Accidents of history created U.S. health system [Radio broadcast episode]. In C. Turpin (Executive Producer), *All Things Considered.* Washington, DC: National Public Radio. Retrieved from http://www.npr.org/templates/story/story.php?storyId=114045132

Cartwright, M.M. (2012, February 20). The high incidence of post Intensive Care Unit (ICU) anxiety and depression. *Psychology Today.* Retrieved from http://www.psychologytoday.com/blog/food-thought/201202/the-high-incidence-post-intensive-care-unit-icu-anxiety-and-depression

Center to Advance Palliative Care, National Palliative Care Research Center. (2011). America's care of serious illness: A state-by-state report card on access to palliative care in our nation's hospitals. Retrieved from http://www.capc.org/reportcard/summary

Centers for Medicare & Medicaid Services. (2013a). CMS covers 100 million people . . . Retrieved from http://www.cms.gov

Centers for Medicare & Medicaid Services. (2013b). How does the health care law protect me? Retrieved from http://www.healthcare.gov/law/features/rights/bill-of-rights/index.html

Centers for Medicare & Medicaid Services. (2013c). Medicaid. Retrieved from http://www.medicare.gov/your-medicare-costs/help-paying-costs/medicaid/medicaid.html

Centers for Medicare & Medicaid Services. (2013d). Medicare. Retrieved from http://www.medicare.gov/your-medicare-costs/help-paying-costs/medicaid/medicaid.html

Centers for Medicare & Medicaid Services. (2013e). Nursing facilities. Retrieved from http://www.medicaid.gov/Medicaid-CHIP-Program-Information/By-Topics/Delivery-Systems/Institutional-Care/Nursing-Facilities-NF.html

Centers for Medicare & Medicaid Services. (2013f). What are the different types of health insurance? Retrieved from https://www.healthcare.gov/what-are-the-different-types-of-health-insurance/

Clancy, C.M. (2008, March-April). How patient-centered healthcare can improve quality. *Patient Safety & Quality Healthcare.* Retrieved from http://www.psqh.com/marapr08/ahrq.html

Clark, K. (2011). The collaborative continuum associated with adverse medical events. *International Journal of Collaborative Practices, 2*(1), 1–11.

Committee on Quality of Health Care in America, Institute of
   Medicine. (1999). *To err is human: Building a safer
   health system.* Washington, DC: The National
   Academies Press. Retrieved from http://iom.edu/
   Reports/1999/To-Err-is-Human-Building-A-Safer-Health-
   System.aspx

Committee on Quality of Health Care in America, Institute of
   Medicine. (2001). *Crossing the quality chasm: A new
   healthcare system for the 21st century.* Washington, DC:
   The National Academies Press. [A summary of the full
   text is available at http://www.iom.edu/Reports/
   2001/Crossing-the-Quality-Chasm-A-New-Health-
   System-for-the-21st-Century.aspx]

Conway, J., Federico, F., Stewart, K., & Campbell, M.J. (2010).
   *Respectful management of serious clinical adverse
   events* (2nd edition). [IHI Innovation Series white paper.
   ] Cambridge, MA: Institute for Healthcare Improvement. Retrieved from http://www.ihi.org/
   knowledge/Pages/IHIWhitePapers/Respectful
   ManagementSeriousClinicalAEsWhitePaper.aspx

Curtin, L. (2012). Forgive us our trespasses. *American Nurse
   Today, 5*(5), 56.

Curtis, D. (2010, July). Sometimes, an apology can deter a
   lawsuit. *California Bar Journal.* Retrieved from
   http://www.calbarjournal.com/July2010/TopHeadlines/
   TH1.aspx

Davis, K., Schoen, C., & Stremikis, K. (2010, June). Mirror,
mirror on the wall: How the performance of the U.S.
health care system compares internationally, 2010
update. [Published by The Commonwealth Fund.]
Retrieved from http://www.commonwealthfund.org/
Publications/Fund-Reports/2010/Jun/Mirror-Mirror-
Update.aspx?page=all

Delbanco, T., Berwick, D.M., Boufford, J.I., Edgman-Levitan, S.,
Ollenschläger, G., Plamping, D., & Rockefeller, R.G.
(2001). Healthcare in a land called PeoplePower: Nothing about me without me. *Health Expectations, 4*(3),
44–50.

Frydman, G. (2013). Patient-driven: The growing impact of
networked patients. Retrieved from
http://www.patientdriven.org/

Health Resources and Services Administration, U.S. Department of Health and Human Services. (2013). HRSA.
Retrieved from http://www.hrsa.gov/index.html

Healthcare Economics and Management. (2009, November 1).
The history of medical insurance in the United States.
*Yale Journal of Medicine & Law: An Undergraduate
Publication.* Retrieved from
http://www.yalemedlaw.com/2009/11/the-history-of-
medical-insurance-in-the-united-states/

Huntington, B., & Kuhn, N. (2003). Communication gaffes: A
root cause of malpractice claims. *Baylor University
Medical Center Proceedings, 16*(2), 157–161. Retrieved
from http://www.ncbi.nlm.nih.gov/pmc/articles/
PMC1201002/

Joint Commission. (2008). Sentinel event alert, issue 40: Behaviors that undermine a culture of safety. Retrieved from http://www.jointcommission.org/sentinel_event_alert_issue_40_behaviors_that_undermine_a_culture_of_safety/

Joint Commission. (2012). Patient safety. Retrieved from http://www.jointcommission.org/topics/patient_safety.aspx

Joint Commission. (2013a). About the Joint Commission. Retrieved from http://www.jointcommission.org/about_us/about_the_joint_commission_main.aspx

Joint Commission. (2013b). National patient safety goals. Retrieved from http://www.jointcommission.org/standards_information/npsgs.aspx

Kenny, L. (2013, April 5). *Addressing the emotional side when things go wrong*. PowerPoint slides presented at Medically Induced Trauma Support Services, Inc., 9th Annual Maryland Patient Safety Conference, Baltimore. Medically Induced Trauma Support Services, Inc. Retrieved from http://www.marylandpatientsafety.org/documents/AnnualConference2013/Track-4-Kenney-PPT-2.pdf

Longo, J. (2010, January 31). Combating disruptive behaviors: Strategies to promote a healthy work environment. *OJIN: The Online Journal of Issues in Nursing, 15*(1), Manuscript 5.

MetLife Mature Market Institute. (2010). *The MetLife study of working caregivers and employer health care costs: New insights and innovations for reducing health care costs for employers.* New York: Author. Retrieved from https://www.metlife.com/assets/cao/mmi/publications/studies/2011/mmi-caregiving-costs-working-caregivers.pdf

Mosby's Medical Dictionary (8th ed.). (2008). Maryland
Heights, MO: Elsevier Health Services.

Murray, C.J., & Frenk, J. (2010, January 14). Ranking 37th—
Measuring the performance of the U.S. health care system. *New England Journal of Medicine, 362,* 98–99.

National Alliance for Caregiving in collaboration with AARP.
(2009). Caregiving in the U.S.: Executive summary.
[Funded by MetLife Foundation.]
Retrieved from http://www.caregiving.org/data/
CaregivingUSAllAgesExecSum.pdf

National Hospice and Palliative Care Organization. (2012).
NHPCO facts and figures: Hospice care in America. Retrieved from http://www.nhpco.org/sites/default/files/
public/Statistics_Research/2012_Facts_Figures.pdf

Oxford Dictionary of English. (2010). New York: Oxford University Press. Retrieved from
http://oxforddictionaries.com/us/definition/
american_english/survival

Rosenstein, A.H., & O'Daniel, M. (2008). A survey of the impact of disruptive behaviors and communication defects
on patient safety. *The Joint Commission Journal on
Quality and Patient Safety, 34*(8), 464–471.

Torrey, T. (2013, February 10). Proactive survivorship—
The sixth stage of grief, a catharsis for anger.
Retrieved from http://patients.about.com/od/
medicalmistakessafety/a/Proactive-Survivorship-The-
Sixth-Stage-Of-Grief.htm

Unresolved disrespectful behavior in healthcare: Practitioners
speak up (again)—Part I. (2013, June 27). *ISMP medication safety alert!* [acute care edition, Institute for Safe

Medication Practices]. Retrieved from
http://www.ismp.org/newsletters/acutecare/
showarticle.aspx?id=52

Weckmann, M.T. (2008). The role of the family physician in
the referral and management of hospice patients. *American Family Physician, 77*(6), 807–812.

World Health Organization. (2013). World health report 2013:
Research for universal health coverage. Retrieved from
http://www.who.int/whr/en/

ABOUT THE AUTHOR

Ruth A. Tarantine, DNP, RN, has been a nurse for 25 years. She has spent the majority of her career working in intensive care units at various hospitals across the country. Although she loves teaching patients and caring for patients at the bedside, she found that she could directly improve the quality of care of many patients through nursing education. Teaching future nurses and future nurse educators is her passion. To this end, she obtained her Doctorate in Nursing Practice in 2008 and began a full-time teaching position at a private university shortly thereafter.

Ruth has presented research nationally and internationally on the use of simulation in health care provider education and its effect on quality of care.

Ruth is also passionate about the care of elders. The experience of navigating the health care system for her mother served as a wakeup call. She was disillusioned with the care of elders she witnessed and vowed to help those that couldn't help themselves.

Ruth started Eldercare Navigators, LLC, with her attorney brother, Rick. Together, they assist elders and chronically ill individuals to navigate the complex health and legal maze. Ironically, they both found that their professions complement each other in the elder community. While elders may face a myriad of medical decisions, they also need legal guidance to protect their assets and plan for their future.

Eldercare Navigators, LLC, offers individual customized health and legal navigation services as well as works with employers to provide elder care benefits to employees who may be caring for aging parents.

To contact Ruth Tarantine with questions about *Against All Odds*, or to inquire about elder navigation services:

Book Website	www.HealthCareAgainstAllOdds.com
Book Inquiries	Info@HealthCareAgainstAllOdds.com
Email	Ruth@HealthCareAgainstAllOdds.com
LinkedIn	www.linkedin.com/in/RuthTarantine
Facebook	https://www.facebook.com/ healthcareagainstallodds
Eldercare Navigators, LLC	www.ElderNavigators.com

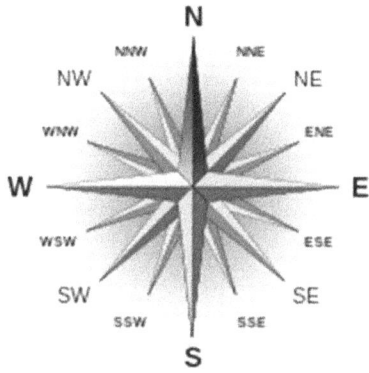

**ELDERCARE
NAVIGATORS, LLC**

www.ingramcontent.com/pod-product-compliance
Lightning Source LLC
Chambersburg PA
CBHW031153270326
41931CB00006B/255